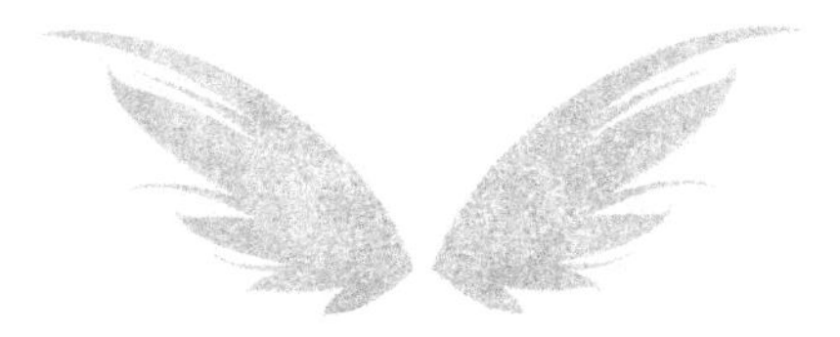

LIVING WITH CANCER

Jonathan's Way

A story of faith, courage and hope

V C Quinn

BJP

First published in Great Britain in 2018 by
Blue-Jay Press

Living with Cancer: *Jonathan's Way*

Cover and interior designs by John Bigwood

ISBN: 978-1-5272-2938-9

2 4 6 8 10 9 7 5 3 1

For Jonathan: my proud and fearless lion.

Also for N, S & N who will always miss him.

AUTHOR'S NOTE

Jonathan's courage helped me to release my own fears about death
and dying. His suffering brought me a spiritual awakening that
I was not prepared for. Above all, his selfless love gave me comfort
and hope when I could find none elsewhere.
I pray his story will do the same for you.

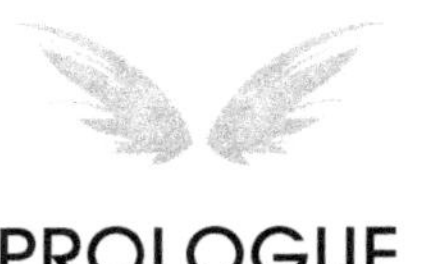

PROLOGUE

'Johnny Angel'

1

February, 1985: I HAD NO IDEA I WAS PREGNANT. A hot tear rolled down my cheek. It splashed onto the pale embryo that lay flat in the palm of my hand. Two black dots – like spots of coal – stared back at me from inside the large head that gently curved into a thick mass of soft scrambled jelly. I scrutinized its translucent spinal column before finally resting the tip of my little finger over my dead baby's heart. It felt warm and sticky. A sharp pain stabbed into the pit of my stomach. I groaned. A sudden gush of bright-red blood trickled down my inner-thighs, soaking the white pedestal mat on which I was standing. A child's painful scream penetrated the windowless bathroom. And I soon panicked when I remembered Richard whom I had left unattended for far too long. A second almighty scream echoed inside my head. Without hesitating, I wrapped my dead baby inside some clean tissue and flushed it down the toilet. Hurriedly tidying myself, I raced out of the bathroom to tend my first born, himself just nine months old. But, to my dismay, guilt chased after me: *Stop worrying*! I told myself. *Nature has done the right thing and so have you*!

However, nature had an even bigger surprise in store on that cold February morning, just days after my twenty-fifth birthday. A truly magnificent surprise I could never have envisaged in a month of Sundays. Indeed, nothing in this world could have prepared me for the happy, yet unexpected, event that was to follow exactly six months later.

2

18ᵗʰ August, 1985: "HOW LONG ARE YOUR CONTRACTIONS?" enquired the Irish midwife, the instant I fell through the delivery suite doors of the Greenwich District Hospital, south east London. It was a hot and humid Sunday, a short time after midnight.

"Long enough to beg for a caesarean!" I gasped, humorously.

But the tiny midwife did not smile. Instead, she calmly led me into a small, sterile room that had a well-worn armchair at one end; a make-shift bed at the other; and a clear Perspex cot in the far, right-hand corner that was fully prepared for the arrival of my unborn baby.

The comforting smell of antiseptic dashed into my nostrils. I inhaled deeply. Glancing past my plump reflection that filled the undressed window opposite, I admired the spectacular view that stretched for miles across historic Greenwich. Like bright birthday candles, hundreds of burning street lamps illuminated the dimmed houses that were sleeping in the silent streets below, whilst the murky river Thames softly rolled towards the City. My dreamy gaze drifted towards the navy sky.

"Wow!" I gasped, when I suddenly felt strangely blessed by the striking mass of silver stars that were dazzling in the heavens like millions of uncut diamonds.

Shuffling my heavy bulk across the spotless floor, I

carefully lowered myself into the old armchair.

"Hello again," I foolishly chuckled to the large cylinder of gas and air that stood soldier-like beside me. Another sharp pain rendered me powerless. The nimble midwife dashed to my side. Holding my limp wrist between her icy fingers, she expertly timed the exact length of my contraction.

"Right!" She cheerfully announced the second it was over. "Now let's take a quick peep on the inside."

Heaving myself out of the comfy chair, I closely observed the meticulous midwife whose beady-blue eyes were now scanning a cold-metal tray filled with shiny utensils.

"Don't reckon I'll be needing an enema!" I tried to joke again, whilst staggering across the dust-free floor. "I've taken enough caster-oil to flush out an army!" I naively continued.

"To be sure, who told you to take that?" enquired the midwife.

Her frosty manner surprised me.

"Oh, a good friend. She said it would get fings moving an' it's certainly done that!"

There was an uncomfortable silence. Her sharp eyes tightened. Hauling myself onto the narrow bed, I shuddered beneath the diligent midwife's disapproving glare.

"We simply don't like that sort of thing anymore. To be sure, it's much kinder for baby to arrive in his own time and not in ours. Don't you think?"

There was another uncomfortable silence. Believing I

had committed a serious offence against my unborn child, my head hung in shame. However, I soon became concerned, once again, when the starchy midwife reached into a small cardboard box and promptly pulled out two vinyl gloves. Skilfully, she tweaked each armoured finger into shape.

"But I'm a week overdue! *And* I've got annuver child to fink of!" I gulped, loudly.

"Now you just relax there, Vicki." She coolly commanded. "This won't take a moment."

I gritted my teeth and tried to obey.

"To be sure, baby is doing well. But not quite ready yet." She eventually told me.

Her pinched face finally cracked into a lovely smile. Regardless, scared by a nagging doubt that had slowly crept into the back of my mind I struggled to regain my composure. Indeed, apart from feeling utterly selfish for putting my own needs above those of my unborn child, I now questioned my ability to cope with the imminent birth. My worried gaze drifted towards the wide window. A beautiful bright-orange light flickered in the distance. Mesmerised, I followed the dancing glow until it completely disappeared. The midwife's flat reflection suddenly stopped beside me.

"Well, isn't that a pretty sight?" Her lyrical voice cooed into the warm summer night.

I fake smiled. She instantly busied herself around the room.

"Now, to be sure." She thoughtlessly continued.

"Would you like me to draw those curtains?"

"*Err*, no fanks!" I bluntly retorted.

"Well, in that case, I'll be leaving you in peace." She happily concluded.

And with that, her blue silhouette finally disappeared behind the heavy hospital door. I breathed a huge sigh of relief. At last I was alone. Flinging my fat arms around my tight belly, I hugged my unborn child for a long time. Then, to my dismay, sudden and vivid flashbacks from Richard's recent birth unexpectedly raced through my mind. I panicked. Especially when I recalled the traumatic pain no-one ever dares to speak about: not even a mother or best friend. My weary eyes darted about the sterile room. They lingered on the large cylinder of gas and air. And when a powerful and inexplicable urge to deliver my second child single-handedly overwhelmed me, my independent mind quickly reasoned: *This is **my** baby an' **my** pain and I ain't having no drugs or monitors this time 'round — that's for sure!*

I soon hatched a plan. Dragging myself off the narrow bed, I routinely paced up and down the cold floor like a deranged mad woman. And my plan worked like magic. Before long, my contractions were coming and going as fast as I could say *gas an' air*! I was delighted.

Also to my delight, the silver stars were still sparkling brightly in the deep-navy sky when the tiny midwife returned to check on my progress. But this time I was pleased to see her. She gasped loudly when she discovered me still standing by the window. Her flat-black shoes raced towards me when I sucked too deeply into the plastic mask and almost stumbled.

"I ... can ... feel ... a head." I wheezed, painfully.

Holding my outstretched arms, the compassionate midwife led me back towards the narrow bed. But I could no longer lift my feet off the ground.

"Don't move!" she ordered, before dashing out of the room to find assistance.

She returned a few moments later with a much larger midwife who easily hoisted me back onto the bed. However, their raucous laughter at the sight of my hygienic paper knickers infuriated me.

"A bit late for those!" teased the larger midwife, heartily.

Then she roughly removed them. But when she proceeded to tug on the cylinder of gas and air due to its excessive use, my misshapen hand gripped the plastic mask very tightly:

"*Please* don't take it away!" I pleaded into her shiny round face that was grinning into mine like a fat Cheshire cat. "I *really* can't cope wivout it!"

Yet the sly midwife continued to massage my crooked hand believing that I was unaware of her trickery.

"I'LL FUCKING *KILL* YOU!" I roared at her, when my grip almost loosened.

Her horrified face instantly retreated to the foot of the bed where her help was more urgently needed.

"STOP PUSHING!" yelled the smaller midwife,

suddenly. "We have big shoulders!"

And in that exact moment, I truly believed I would die from the pain that was ripping me apart.

"Stop push ..."

The midwife's insistent voice faded into a hazy echo. I awoke to the sound of squeaky tyres being wheeled across a hard floor. And when the soothing mask unexpectedly leapt out of my gnarled hand and bounced across the room, I seethed with anger and frustration because I was unable to chase after it.

"Stay awake!" commanded the smaller midwife. "Your baby *needs* you!"

"It sodding *hurts*!" I screeched at her. "It *really* hurts!"

"I *know* it hurts, dear." She calmly quipped. "But not for much longer. To be sure, do you want to feel your baby's head?"

I opened my mouth to screech once more but no sound came out. Helplessly defeated, my hot head sank into the stiff-white pillows.

Nonetheless, my stubborn mind urged me to remain strong. *After all*, I reminded myself: *this is **my** baby and **my** pain*! And so, at precisely 03.51a.m. I astounded the ponderous midwives when I defiantly pushed my baby into this world regardless of whether the timing was right or not.

3

HOW I LOVED MY SECOND SON the instant I held him in my arms. "Hello, cute little man," I affectionately whispered into his teeny-tiny ear whilst brushing his downy cheek against mine. His soft, warm skin smelt like sweet honeycomb. And the pleasing pull of his tight grip tugging on my own finger was equally comforting. Our eyes locked for a long time. Oddly, I felt his sharp, intense gaze already knew me. For sure, he looked a lot like me. He was alert too, becoming easily distracted by the noisy midwives who were genuinely surprised by his long, muscular frame that weighed-in at nine pounds one ounce.

"But his feet and legs are crooked!" I whined to the tiny midwife, approximately one hour later. "*And* he still ain't cried yet!"

She tried to reassure me.

"He just needs a good stretch. Gently massage his soft bones over the next few days and he'll soon straighten."

"Seriously, though, shouldn't we be smacking him or summink?"

"No, really. He's grand: just happy and contented. To be sure, I'd pray he stayed that way if it were me!"

I held my precious bundle very tightly as the porter wheeled us to the maternity ward a few hours later. Everything felt right as we sailed through the empty corridors of the Greenwich District, passing the double lifts and chapel on the way. I closed my eyes. And for the first time since his delivery, I pondered on a suitable name for my unusually serene son. Then, from nowhere, the name *Jonathan* leapt into my tired mind. It sounds absurd, I know, but I was truly surprised because I had never once thought of it before. *But he'll get called John an' that's just boring!* I inwardly argued. Yet

Jonathan continued to crowd my sleepy thoughts. *You could name him J.J. for short*, I cheerfully concluded: *J.J. Yep. I really like that!*

Nevertheless, I still tried to think of a more preferable name. But the harder I tried the louder I heard *Jonathan* resounding inside my head. So that by the time we reached the maternity ward I was fully convinced 'Jonathan' was, indeed, a fine name for a fine son.

Of course, my family and friends were as surprised as I was by my unexpected name choice. But I told no-one about its inspiration. And when I searched through my book of Babies Names the instant I arrived home and discovered that 'Jonathan' means 'a gift from God' then, naturally, I could not argue with that.

4

JONATHAN WAS FIVE YEARS OLD when my marriage to his father ended in divorce. He remained my quietest child who rarely spoke unless he had something intelligent to say. Furthermore, in addition to Richard he now also had Daniel, aged three, and Rosie, aged one, to contend with. Unsurprisingly, most evenings inside our lively Woolwich Common abode ended with someone in tears, usually Daniel. But canny Jonathan soon learnt to play alone - and in complete silence - until his much noisier siblings were peacefully tucked-up in bed. Only then would he emerge from his inconspicuous corner to join me downstairs for a nice cup of tea with ginger-nut biscuit. And, of course, I saw no harm in indulging my second son – who still looked a lot like me - with some of the quality time he so obviously needed.

I recall when Jonathan was much younger and how our evening get-togethers always began with his favourite bedtime story, entitled *The Proud and Fearless Lion*. It's a delightful story about a majestic lion that becomes sick and subsequently sleeps through the entrapment of his fellow companions by a greedy circus owner. However, the proud and fearless lion eventually saves the day when he frightens the circus owner out of the jungle with a magnificent roar that proves him truly worthy of his title as King of the Jungle. "ROAR!" Jonathan always bellowed at this point in the story. And, in a surprised tone, I would always say: "Oh my goodness, Jonathan. You sounded just like a real lion when you did that!" Then, without fail, Jonathan would screw-up his tiny, lion-like face before producing another much louder roar that would cause us to fall about with laughter.

Before long, 'Jonny's Time' became an evening ritual that we both enjoyed very much. As he grew, I delighted in his intelligent wit and brilliant sense of humour. Whilst he revelled in listening to my sentimental stories from his early years, especially the one in which he refused to sleep until I sung 'Johnny Angel' over and over again into his teeny baby ear. "Seriously, Jon. You blinking wore me out!" I often concluded, which always highly amused him. Then sometimes, just for fun, Jonathan would plead with me to sing him his special song once more. Of course, I always did.

In truth, Jonathan never outgrew our evening chats together mostly because apart from our looks we also shared remarkably similar personalities too. And so naturally, an extra-strong and special bond instinctively formed between us.

LIVING WITH CANCER
Jonathan's Way

A story of faith, courage and hope

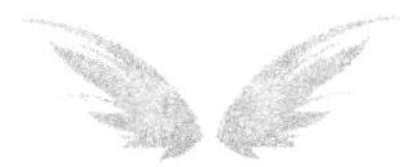

ACT ONE

Faith

'No man was ever wise by chance'

(- Seneca)

Characters

JONATHAN JAMES, aged fifteen years. Tall and slim; Large, hazel eyes; and short, light-brown hair. Honest, intelligent and wise. JONATHAN is unafraid to express his profound views on death and dying.

RICHARD (his brother), aged sixteen years. Medium height and build; large, dark-brown eyes; and short, light-brown hair. Gentle and polite.

DANIEL (his brother), aged twelve years. Tall and slim; large, dark-brown eyes; and short, dark-brown hair. Emotional and shy.

ROSIE (his sister) aged ten years. Above average height; dark-brown eyes; and long, dark-brown hair. Sensible and considerate.

VICKI (their mother), early forties. Below average height. Green-blue eyes; and short, dark-blonde hair. Realistic and assertive. Her direct manner is frequently misunderstood by others. Like her children, she has a strong, south London accent.

CAROLINE, Producer/Director/Interviewer employed by the BBC. Small and petite; large, light-blue eyes; and long, light-blonde hair. She has a standard, British television accent.

JACK, Cameraman employed by the BBC. Extremely tall; sharp-blue eyes; and cropped, dark-brown hair. He has a soft, well-educated British accent.

MAX, Sound engineer employed by the BBC. Medium height and build; dark-brown eyes; and short, light-brown hair. He has a pleasing, upper-class British accent.

Setting: A three bedroom semi on a small south London council estate.

Additional Note: Because this prose drama is a true story, all of the character's names except JONATHAN and VICKI have been changed to protect their identities.

SCENE ONE

7th February, 2001: *It is 7.00 a.m. VICKI (wearing a long-sleeve, lilac tee-shirt; black trousers; and white trainers) is kneeling on top of her tidied, four-poster bed. Through half-opened curtains, she is observing CAROLINE, JACK, and MAX who are discussing area shots on the empty street below. The big, brass bed - that fills most of the floor space inside her cosy box-room - has a set of white rosary beads loosely entwined around the left post. A small, bronze crucifix hangs on the wall beside them. Although the black floor lamp to VICKI's right is switched on, its dim glow barely lifts the early morning darkness. Continuing clockwise, a slim, black bookcase crammed with old Disney videos; Penguin classics; and self-help/spiritual books fills the tiny gap at the foot of the bed. A similar bookcase rests against the adjacent wall directly opposite the window, along with a full-length, gold-rimmed mirror. An in-built linen cupboard is to the door right. And some white chest-of- drawers occupy the remaining floor space, door left. A large, purple teddy sits at the foot of the bed. It matches the vibrant purple and gold wallpaper; the duvet set; and the half-opened curtains. Lastly, every shelf, unit and ledge inside this cramped, yet relaxed, bedroom overflows with a variety of family photographs; much-loved music c.ds; and everyday cosmetics. The sun is almost fully risen. But daylight is struggling to break through the dark, menacing clouds that are racing across the wintry sky. Suddenly, a middle-aged workman appears on the rain-stained pavement that is glistening beneath two burning streetlamps. He coughs loudly; crosses the crescent; then swiftly disappears into the hazy distance. And the rumbling roar from the nearby A2 motorway - that has been faintly reverberating throughout- gradually rises before merging with the sharp, energetic shrill coming from some invisible bird life. Together, they challenge the strong, howling wind for precedence over the brand new day. (VICKI speaks to the camera that Jack has left running inside her bedroom doorway):*

IT ALL BEGAN AROUND MARCH, 1999. Jonathan was thirteen years old when a small swelling appeared inside the arch of his left foot. Naturally, he complained about some pain but only a little. And, of course, when he told me about the particularly bad football injury he sustained just a few weeks earlier, we both believed his sore foot would heal by itself over time as these types of injuries so often did. Anyhow, approximately ten weeks passed. Early one Saturday evening, feeling more than excited about our forthcoming trip to the Isle of Wight, the children and I huddled together inside our tiny front-room as we waited to watch *Noel's House Party* on the television. I turned to Jonathan who was sitting close beside me on our shabby-pink sofa:

"Fetch me yer cream from the bathroom, Jon. I may as well do yer feet while we're sitting 'ere." I casually said, knowing the hot sand would destroy the soles of his feet due to eczema.

However, when Jonathan saw Richard mischievously grinning in our direction he soon became reluctant to do as I asked.

"He'll take my seat! I know he will!" He noisily protested.

"No he won't, Jon! I promise." I firmly insisted. "Now go fetch that cream!"

And so on, after much fuss, Jonathan did as I asked. Of course, we all roared with laughter when Richard instantly leapt into Jonathan's vacant seat the moment he left the room.

"You betta be outta there as soon as I get back!" Jonathan growled at his older brother, whilst bolting up the stairs. And, naturally, I forced Richard out of Jonathan's prized seat the moment he returned. Re-settled beside me, Jonathan carefully removed his socks:

"Oh yeah, mum. You can see how big that lump's got," he

coolly remarked, before dropping his left foot into the centre of my lap. "See how weird it looks," he continued. "And it's still *very* painful!"

Richard, Daniel, and Rosie quickly gathered around us. And, together, we scrutinized Jonathan's left foot for a long time.

"Ooh, it *does* look painful." Daniel eventually sympathised.

"Mum. I'm telling yer: that ain't blinking normal!" declared Richard, adamantly.

Jonathan frowned. Whilst I remained silently puzzled by the large, solid lump that entirely filled the inside of his left foot. Indeed, I was truly stunned by how rapid the small swelling had grown since March. Also to my horror, the hot, pulsating lump was beginning to spread beneath the base of Jonathan's toes and starting to poke through the top of his foot via the metatarsal bones.

"Bloody hell, Jonny!" I finally screeched. "Why haven't you shown me this sooner?"

But Jonathan remained perfectly silent. Regardless, we arrived at our local hospital within the hour. And yet, to my surprise, a thorough x-ray failed to confirm my own suspicion that a broken bone had to be entirely responsible for the abnormal swelling inside Jonathan's left foot. And although the bewildered doctor agreed that the swelling was unusually large, he promptly diagnosed a stress fracture and insisted that it would heal by itself over time.

Two days passed. The children were having a fantastic time playing together on the sandy Isle of Wight beach, whilst I reclined in my deck chair closely observing Jonathan's obvious limp from beneath my over-sized sunglasses. Indeed, because his inability to walk comfortably was becoming more noticeable by the day, I decided an urgent visit to our doctor was in order the instant we returned home.

Two weeks passed. Like us, Doctor N was greatly perplexed by the large swelling inside Jonathan's left foot. He agreed it looked abnormal. However, he also agreed with the doctor at our local hospital and reassured us that a latent stress fracture was the most likely cause. But "to be on the safe side" Doctor N requested a full blood test to check Jonathan's auto-immune system was in order. He also wanted to rule out the rare possibility that he was suffering from gout. Anyhow, at the same time, Doctor N arranged for Jonathan to see a physiotherapist who - after watching him walk up and down a corridor a few times - glibly told us that he was suffering from "Reflex Dystrophy Syndrome" which was undoubtedly caused by his earlier football injury. And to this day, I thank God - for some inexplicable reason - we did not attend her immediate appointment for Jonathan to receive some ultra-sound treatment that she said would help to "break down the swelling".

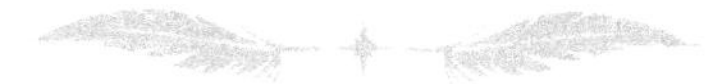

SCENE TWO

It is 8.00 a.m. JACK*'s bulky camera is now standing in the near,
left-hand corner of* VICKI*'s small front-room in which the light-green
wallpaper is fading and the dull-white doors are extensively chipped.
A carriage clock; a bronze crucifix; and a couple of pink birthday cards
sit on top of the wide, old-fashioned gas heater that dominates the
central wall. Moving clockwise, a framed photograph of* JONATHAN
*shaking hands with Pope John Paul 11; a bowl of mixed fruit; and two
more birthday cards crowd the round coffee table situated near the
gas heater. An early photograph of the children and two more birthday
cards are on top of the heavy, stone-grey television that consumes the
far, right-hand corner. A red bean-bag sits in the centre of the big bay-
window. Several more photographs of the children and two pot plants
adorn the red-stone window-ledge. The distorted metal window-frames
are disguised beneath some crisp-white netting. A pair of olive-green
curtains match the cheap, acrylic carpet perfectly. But the broad,
pink and blue rug in the centre of the room adds some much needed
colour. A shabby-pink sofa with mismatched cushions runs along the
right, nearside wall. And a large, mahogany dining-table with six
sturdy chairs fills the entire left-hand corner. Six table mats; a bowl of
oranges; a carton of fruit juice; a jar of raspberry jam; a jar of peanut
butter; a plate of buttered toast; and a pretty vase of red carnations
have been strategically placed upon it. Finally, a wild elephant print;
a large flower print; and a colourful picture of Jesus Christ with the
words 'I Trust in You' inscribed beneath it adorn the interior walls of
this busy, family orientated front-room.*

All of the characters, except RICHARD, *are prepared for
some in-house filming that* CAROLINE *has arranged for the purpose
of her BBC 'Cancer' documentary. However, unknown to her, this
simple family scene is somewhat contrived because in reality the
residents at 228, Linklow Crescent hardly ever start their day at the*

"

same time let alone sit together for early morning breakfast. At the moment when filming begins, JONATHAN (casually dressed in his favourite blue jumper and jeans) is resting his head face down upon the dining table. ROSIE (wearing a blue school blouse and navy skirt) is seated beside him. CAROLINE is seated on the shabby- pink sofa. MAX – holding a fur-covered microphone high into the air - is standing behind JACK who is kneeling behind his tripod and camera. And VICKI and DANIEL (wearing a white school shirt, grey trousers, and burgundy blazer) are busy preparing breakfast in the adjacent kitchen. (VICKI speaks to camera):

MEANWHILE, I TOOK JONATHAN TO see Doctor N several more times during August to December. And, naturally, I trusted in his professional opinion when he continued to insist that Jonathan's swollen foot was due to a severe stress fracture most likely caused by his earlier football injury. However, because Jonathan's left foot failed to respond to Doctor N's recommended 'hot and cold' water treatment, he kindly sent him for a further blood test; another x-ray; and even an M.R.I. scan. And each time I called the surgery for the test results the efficient receptionist dutifully informed me that they had all come back negative. But Jonathan's left foot continued to grow at a steady rate. Eventually, his foot became so large that he was barely able to walk unaided let alone wear a shoe. The time soon arrived when we had no choice but to ask Doctor N for some crutches so that Jonathan could still attend school -

JONATHAN I've been up since four!

(He quickly lifts his head off the dining-table and sits bolt upright. His gold cross and chain falls loosely around his neck. His pale, young face is neatly framed with short, well-shaped side-burns and a soft mop of wavy-brown hair. A tiny scar cuts into the top of his right eyebrow. Two small moles highlight his left cheek. His lips are neither too thick nor too thin. His slightly protruding ears and wide nostrils balance out

his strong jaw-line perfectly. And his large, hazel eyes appear heavy through lack of sleep. He is clearly anxious at being filmed for the first time because his left knee is habitually bouncing up and down whilst he regularly sips from the small bottle of natural spring water that he carries with him at all times.)

CARO Is that when you wake-up – four o/clock?

JONATHAN Yeah. Bright as a bird!

(The microwave bleeps three times from inside the run-down kitchen that has only a few fitted units; cheap-white netting at the window; and some water damaged linoleum on the cold, concrete floor. A vast number of kitchen utensils and food items are strewn over the work tops, including: coffee, milk, lemonade, bleach, a blackened baking dish, green washing-up liquid and some yellow plastic gloves.)

VICKI *(from kitchen)* Jonathan! – do you want some fruit juice?

JONATHAN *(humorously)* No thank you, Mummy! I'll have some water.

(JONATHAN rises from the dining table and joins VICKI and DANIEL inside the kitchen. VICKI is mixing some warm milk and cereal together inside a small dish. Her looped earrings match her gold cross pendant that is clearly visible from around her neck.)

CARO *(browsing through some recently taken photographs)* Is that picture of you, Jon?

JONATHAN *(re-entering front-room)* Oh, yeah. It is.

CARO It's sweet.

VICKI *(inside doorway)* I'll probably have summa them on the wall next time you come up. *(Fully entering the front-room, she places the small cereal dish onto the dining table.*) Here's your Ready Brek, Rose.

ROSIE Thank you!

(VICKI *returns to the kitchen where she noisily prepares some toast under the grill.*)

(CAROLINE *picks up* JONATHAN*'s favourite photograph.*)

VICKI (*inside doorway*) Isn't that lovely?

CARO It's gorgeous! It's kinda … *thoughtful.*

JONATHAN Yeah. She told me to act like that! She said: "Look at this thing an' act like you're thinking about summink!" I had to *pretend* I was thinking!

CARO (*humorously*) *Pretend* you were thinking? What - there wasn't anything going through your head? (ROSIE *laughs*) How do you *pretend* to think? You think all the time, don't you? I can't imagine you don't ever have thoughts inside your head!

(*Pause*)

JONATHAN *And* I had make-up on my face!

CARO *Did* you? (ROSIE *laughs again*) You girl, you! (*Pause*) They're brilliant. Really, really nice.

(*Long pause.* DANIEL, *who has been secretly hiding inside the kitchen throughout, is finally spotted by* JONATHAN *when he sneaks into the fridge to fetch some milk.*)

JONATHAN (*loudly*) Eat yer breakfast, Dan! You've gotta be there in a minute!

VICKI Dan! At least have some fruit juice. (*She noisily arranges some plates onto the kitchen table and butters the freshly made toast.*)

JONATHAN (*mockingly*) Take a seat, Dan! Don't be shy!

DANIEL (*calmly*) I'm not hungry.

JONATHAN What d'yer mean you're not hungry? That's a first!

(*Long pause.* JONATHAN *softly whistles as he re-takes his seat at the dining table. Suddenly,* RICHARD (*wearing a black, short-sleeved tee-shirt and blue jeans*) *enters the room. His heavy hair is dishevelled and he appears unnaturally pale and sleepy.* JONATHAN *chuckles.*)

JONATHAN (*to* RICHARD) Good morning!

RICHARD (*giving a shy wave to the BBC crew*) Morning. S..s .sorry. (*He attempts to escape into the kitchen.*)

VICKI (*to* RICHARD, *humorously*) Oh, say good morning! Caroline –

CARO It's alright, we've met.

VICKI (*surprised*) Oh, have you met before?

CARO Yeah. We go back a long way! Just pretend we're not here, Rick.

(RICHARD *quickly disappears into the kitchen.*)

JONATHAN (*to* CAROLINE) Don't usually sit-up here and eat like this.

(ROSIE *giggles*)

DANIEL (*finally entering the front-room*) See yer later, mates.

JONATHAN Bye. Oh, yer not late!

(DANIEL *quickly reaches the front-room door.*)

VICKI See yer Dan. What time yer home?

DANIEL I dunno. Whenever.

(VICKI *and* DANIEL *exit the front-room together. They are heard saying goodbye to each other at the front door.* VICKI *returns to the front-room. She sits beside* RICHARD *who is now seated at the dining table.*)

JONATHAN When was the last time we all sat-up here and had breakfast together?

RICHARD Never!

ROSIE (*softly*) It's not difficult!

(*Everyone in the room laughs*)

CARO Just do what you normally do. Don't do things just for us.

JONATHAN (*defiantly*) I'll stick the tele on then!

(JONATHAN *rises from the dining table and sits on the sofa beside* CAROLINE.)

VICKI (*embarrassed*) Jonathan! Sit up here!

JONATHAN (*adamantly*) But that's *not* what I normally do!

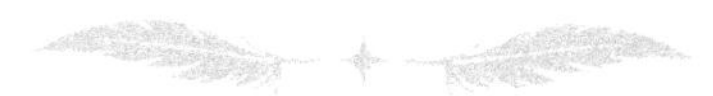

SCENE THREE

It is 10 a.m. RICHARD, DANIEL, *and* ROSIE *have left for school.*
JONATHAN, *wearing the same clothes as earlier, is comfortably
seated on the shabby-pink sofa. The strong, mid-morning sun is shining
brightly through the big bay-window. It highlights the entire right-
hand side of his handsome, young face giving him a soft, ethereal glow
throughout. The vase of red carnations is now situated on the red-stone
window-ledge. A golden ornamental butterfly rests upon a tall pot
stand to* JONATHAN*'s right. And the vibrant picture of Jesus Christ
with the words 'I Trust in You' inscribed beneath it hangs on the wall
directly above his head. As the scene opens,* JACK *is adjusting his
camera in preparation for* JONATHAN*'s first one-to-one interview
with* CAROLINE *who is seated on a dining chair opposite him.
Holding his microphone high,* MAX *is standing behind her. Whilst*
VICKI *is watching a small television screen that has been conveniently
set-up on the kitchen table. (She speaks to camera):*

 IT WAS A DAMP AND dreary mid-December afternoon
when Jonathan - knowing just how unhappy I was with Doctor N - sat
quietly beside me inside the cramped waiting area of his busy surgery.
I grew increasingly tense. At last it was our turn to be seen. Quickly,
I marched straight into Doctor N's consulting room with Jonathan, on
crutches, limping behind me.

 "Take off yer sock!" I ordered, the moment Jonathan had
lowered himself into the chair situated at the side of Doctor N's desk.
I stood behind him, refusing to exchange pleasantries with the popular
young doctor who smiled far too much for my own liking. Instead, I
pointed at Jonathan's left foot and hurriedly said:

 "Now the fing is, Doctor. I can't see how you can keep saying
this is a stress fracture when even *I* know *that* should be getting smaller

by now! It just don't make no sense!"

Doctor N stopped smiling. Staring at me in a highly perplexed manner, he frowned. Stroking his long, pointed chin and leaning forward in his black-leather chair, he then scrutinized Jonathan's left foot as though he were looking at it for the very first time.

"Mmm …" he murmured, in a bewildered tone. "Well, yes. The thing is, according to Jonathan's latest x-ray results it appears he has a broken metatarsal bone in his second toe and *that* has been the cause of your son's problem all along!"

Jonathan spun in his seat. His jaw dropped. And the look of sheer disbelief inside his large, hazel eyes mirrored my own tremendous surprise at the sudden and confident manner in which Doctor N had just delivered his final diagnosis.

"A broken metatarsal bone?" I squeaked.

"Yes. That's right," beamed Doctor N. "Unfortunately, the bones inside the foot are *so* small it's often difficult to detect these types of injuries."

And although extremely upset by Doctor N's delayed diagnosis, I remained silent for Jonathan's sake.

"Oh, well." I eventually sighed. "At least summink positive can now be done to help Jonathan."

"Yeah. An' I can get back to school looking normal again!" he quickly added.

Continuously nodding, Doctor N appeared delighted.

Anyhow, in truth, our spirits were greatly lifted by the time we left Doctor N's surgery on that damp and dreary December afternoon. Indeed, both Jonathan and I were truly elated to finally discover the real cause behind his debilitating injury. In fact, even before leaving his surgery Doctor N had arranged for Jonathan to have his foot set in plaster so that we could drive home happy in the knowledge that he would soon return to school fully fit and well again after the festive season -

JONATHAN Dan and Rosie look similar – don't yer fink?

CARO Yes.

JONATHAN They could pass as twins if Rosie was bigger.

CARO Yeah, they *are* quite similar. (*Then professionally*) So Jonathan, I thought first of all we'd go through some of the stuff from last year and then get to where we are at now. But if you had to describe what this last year has been like for you could you sum it up?

JONATHAN (*jokily*) Erm, what … in a word?

CARO Well, maybe not in *one* word. You know, some people if you said (*lightly*) "What's this last year been like for you?" They'd go, "Ah, you know, it's just been a roller-coaster of ups and downs." I don't know. Could you …?

JONATHAN (*nervously tapping his bottle of natural spring water*) It has been a nightmare. I know that phrase is often used but this actually *has* been a nightmare. It actually seems like yer …

CARO (*slightly agitated*) Sorry. The sound of that. Do you want to put the bottle …?

JONATHAN (*innocently*) Huh? (*Nodding towards the camera*) Is it on? Oh, yeah. Umm, yeah, it actually *has* been a nightmare. I've often thought that I should wake-up an' sort myself out 'cos when I have nightmares I often wanna just go and … I wanna go an' kill myself. I've often felt like that in hospital when I've been a bit, yer know, inside of me … I've been a bit weird. I've just wanted to go out and run in front of a bus an' just get it over and done with. (*Pause*) That's what it's been like. So …

CARO Is that because it's something you kind of think is never going to happen to you?

JONATHAN No, not really. 'Cos when I first thought of the word cancer - before all this - I thought, "Right. Yeah, it's bad." But I actually didn't know anyfing about it so I didn't know *how* bad until I actually had treatment and realised all the different side-effects that there were. There's so many! And so many bad feelings inside of you that it makes it that much worse than you fink it will be. So …

CARO What did cancer mean to you then when you first …

JONATHAN (*quickly*) When I first got told? My reactions were, "Right. I'm *really* surprised that this tumour is malignant and not benign." And the first fing that went into my head was, "Right. He said you're gonna have chemotherapy!" And at first I thought, "Right. I'm gonna lose my hair. And I'm gonna have a couple of pills to get me back on my feet and up an' running again." That's the first fing that come into my head. I thought it wasn't gonna be that bad at all. Until I had my first round of chemotherapy. That's when I realised what it was like. And I saw all the people with their hair missing an' the bags running into their chests an' all that business.

CARO Maybe what you could explain to me, in a brief way, is exactly what kind of cancer you have got and what treatment you've been through. (*Incidentally*) You know, say, "Over the last year you had …"

JONATHAN (*quickly*) Over the last year I've had a sarcoma in my left foot.

CARO Can you explain it?

JONATHAN A soft-tissue sarcoma.

CARO Could you explain that to me?

JONATHAN No.

CARO But just explain what you've got. Say "I was diagnosed with …". Or …

JONATHAN (*quickly*) I was diagnosed with a soft-tissue sarcoma in my foot.

CARO And what was the treatment?

JONATHAN The treatment was, erm, four lots of chemotherapy all together over six courses which lasted about four days each. And then I planned to have an operation after that to get rid of the tumour in my foot what it hadn't got rid of by the chemotherapy. Four lots of chemotherapy, which was *really* potent and *really* strong. That's what I needed to get rid of it.

CARO And do you remember when you first went into 'The Teenager's …

JONATHAN Ahh, I was *so* scared because obviously I didn't know that it would be *this* bad. I thought, "Blimey. Look at all these people: they're *so* ill. Their hair is missing!" That's the first fing that hit me was their hair 'cos it's abnormal to see people with patchy hair. You don't usually see it. And then I was just shocked. I wanted to get outta there! I went into the Dayroom and I saw some boy in there with patchy hair an' he was *really* ill looking. And then it went through my mind: "*I* might have to be in here for ages an' have all that done to me!" (JONATHAN *half laughs*) I didn't stay in there long. I had to get outta there. Me an' my mum went home then.

CARO Because you've never heard of this before was it good to know that there are other people going through …?

JONATHAN (*quickly*) No. I didn't find it was. I found it *harder* to know that other people were going through it because I could see them at different stages further on and I could kinda picture what was gonna happen to me. D'yer know what I mean? I could hear them throwing-up at night. Waking me up, yer know, a couple of beds next to me was like (JONATHAN *mimics the sound of someone vomiting*) WERRGH! I was like, "Oh no, I can't get to sleep 'cos someone's throwing-up!" And I thought, "Christ, is that gonna be me three months down the line?" It's *horrible*. I was completely ignorant about what was gonna happen to me an' what I was gonna go through. So then my mind was just finking about all these other people's situations and what could happen then. "Could it be the same as *that* boy? Could it be the same as *that* girl?" So my mind was like asking me questions that I couldn't answer. So …I didn't know what was in store for me then. I was just guessing an' that was horrible.

CARO And during that time, Jon, when you were first …

JACK (*quietly*) Sorry, Caroline …

CARO (*to* JACK) The sunlight? OK. Let's change tape.

JACK *replaces the used video tape in his camera and the interview between* JONATHAN *and* CAROLINE *recommences from where it left off. All five characters are positioned as before. And the strong, mid-morning sun is still shining brightly through the big bay-window. It continues to highlight the entire right-hand side of* JONATHAN'*s handsome, young face giving him a soft, ethereal glow throughout.* (VICKI *speaks to camera*):

        THE WEEK BEFORE CHRISTMAS, 1999, soon arrived. Inside the cramped Orthopaedic clinic at the Greenwich District

Hospital, Jonathan sat quietly beside me whilst I chatted with an old friend whom I had not seen since his nursery days. He grew bored but, thankfully, the long queue soon lessened. Eventually, Jonathan was just one patient away from treatment when a plump Indian doctor with a jolly-round face carefully stepped over his bare foot that was lazily stretched-out before him.

"Whoops! Sorry, young man," smiled the polite doctor. "And whom might you be waiting to see?" He unexpectedly continued.

Doctor Patel's intense gaze lingered over Jonathan's bare foot. Meanwhile, Jonathan joked with the cheery doctor informing him that after an extremely long wait it would soon be his turn to have his foot set in plaster.

"Mmm …," mused Doctor Patel, thoughtfully. "But before you do anything else might I suggest you first see me in my clinic?" Jonathan frowned at me. "Come on!" encouraged the friendly doctor when he saw that we did not wish to lose our place in the queue.

And so, I reluctantly handed Jonathan his crutches and walked behind him as he tottered into Doctor Patel's clinic. He lowered himself into the chair situated at the side of his desk. I stood behind him, closely observing the light-hearted doctor as he intently read through Jonathan's medical notes. Then Doctor Patel examined his foot in the same attentive manner. Finally, the thorough doctor asked us an array of questions that we were used to answering by now:

"So when did the lump first appear?" He began.

"Mid-August." Jonathan and I replied in unison. "But …" Jonathan continued, "It's *really* been there since about last March - only much smaller. I had a bad football injury where annuver player jumped *so* hard – see, just there. "

Jonathan pointed to the exact spot where a rival football player had jumped onto the top of his foot with such force that his studs pricked through the leather of Jonathan's boot and even his sock. Doctor Patel looked astonished.

"And how long have you needed the crutches?" He asked, sympathetically.

"Erm, say from about the last six weeks." Jonathan pondered.

He turned to me for reassurance. I nodded. Then, to my complete surprise, Doctor Patel casually asked me:

"And is Jonathan your only son, Mrs James?"

Initially, I was thrown by his irrelevant question. But because the kind doctor seemed sincere, I quickly reasoned there was no harm in telling him that Jonathan had two brothers and one sister.

"My goodness! You don't look old enough!" He predictably joked.

But I did not laugh. Instead, I became increasingly suspicious and confused by Doctor Patel's jovial, yet highly professional, manner. In my mind, something did not quite add up. Yet I could not easily pin-point the problem. And so, for Jonathan's sake, I remained silent. However, when Doctor Patel proceeded to telephone the ultra-sound department and then personally escorted us there for Jonathan's immediate appointment, I secretly wondered if Doctor N could have possibly, once again, misdiagnosed Jonathan's crippling injury.

"Can Jonathan have his foot set in plaster now?" I impatiently asked Doctor Patel, the instant we returned to his clinic.

"Jonathan will need some more blood tests *plus* another chest x-ray before ..."

"But his broken toe, Doctor? The clinic will close soon!"
I persisted.

"Mrs James. Jonathan does *not* have a broken toe …"

"What d'yer mean no broken toe? Doctor N said …"

Doctor Patel's shiny-black head dropped. He stared vacantly
into Jonathan's medical notes. My heart raced. And when I caught
sight of Jonathan's large, hazel eyes that were staring up at me from his
seat, I almost wept for my sick son who was clearly exhausted due to a
severe flu virus. Anyhow, within minutes, Doctor Patel had telephoned
both the Radiology and Pathology departments requesting for Jonathan
to have some further tests: and all in that same afternoon.

"So what *has* Jonathan got?" I finally asked the efficient
doctor, the instant he put down his telephone.

"Well … it's difficult to say," he ruminated, before continuing
in a more cheery manner: "But someone will contact you once we have
received today's results, which should only take about a week."

"So he ain't got no stress fracture?"

"No."

"An' we'll know in about a week?"

"Yes."

"But …"

Once again, Jonathan's large, hazel eyes were staring up at
me. And I grew instantly silent when his flushed face told me just how
tired he had become by the day's unexpected events. Nevertheless,
with the aid of his dependable crutches Jonathan bravely soldiered-on

to both the Radiology and Pathology departments before we finally ventured home -

CARO Jonathan. When you were first told you got cancer did you feel angry?

JONATHAN (*quickly*) No. I didn't feel angry. I just felt shocked. Well, I s'pose later on when I realised what cancer actually entailed and had in store for me – I was angry then. I was angry at my local doctor up the road 'cos he was dismissing it as, erm, (*mockingly*) "a stress fracture", as "possibly arthritis" an' all that. But it wasn't. It works out that it wasn't an' it was summink more sinister. So I s'pose I was angry at him later on when I was feeling *really* ill and I didn't know what was gonna happen. I was angry then, yeah. But not to begin with I wasn't. I was just shocked an' like … couldn't believe it. That's more like it.

CARO Did cancer mean …

JACK (*quietly*) Sorry. I need to do a battery change.

CARO (*to* JACK) OK. (*To* JONATHAN) Really: is that what it was?

JONATHAN Really. Trust me! Honestly! It might sound stupid but that's true.

CARO What: can you explain that? You just thought …

JONATHAN (*quickly*) What: that I thought that when I first got diagnosed I thought I could have a couple of pills an' be off home? That's *exactly* what I thought! I didn't have a clue what was going on.

CARO How old were you, Jonathan?

JONATHAN I was …what was it now? Erm, Christmas ninety … nine, so that was … (JONATHAN *concentrates*) fourteen. Fourteen, I think. Yeah, fourteen. Yeah, that's right.

CARO So you were fourteen years old and someone said: "Right, you've got cancer" and you just didn't know what that meant?

JONATHAN (*shaking his head*) Not at all! I knew it was bad 'cos I've seen summink on the tele about it (JONATHAN *mimics speech*) "Cancer. People moping around all sad" an' all that. So I thought, "Ooh, let's hope I never get that!" Yer know: that type of fing. But I didn't have a clue. I was just *so* stupid!

CARO I don't think it's stupid. I think if you haven't seen it before why *would* you know? I mean, it's not something that usually happens.

JONATHAN Yeah. But it seems stupid now that I know so much about it. I thought, "God, why didn't I know all this before?" How can so much just mean so little to me to begin with?

CARO And once you started realising what it meant - once you got into the hospital - why *did* you feel angry? What was your main thought? Did you think it was unfair that it was you?

JONATHAN Erm … Yeah. I gotta admit I did. 'Cos I thought cancer started with people smoking an' all that. Well, I s'pose it does really – some strands. And I thought, "I'm someone that's never like put a cigarette to my mouth once in my life an' I've got summink like this!" And I thought, "How come this has happened to *me*? There's chain-smokers out there that don't get this!" I just felt *really* gutted. And I was picturing everyone else getting on with their own lives. Going to school; going to work – everyone I knew – an' there's me: my life has just stopped an' just come to a standstill just 'cos … just 'cos this has happened to me. I can't do anyfing. I've just stopped living!

(*The strong sunlight that has been enhancing the entire right-hand side of* JONATHAN*'s handsome, young face throughout suddenly becomes much stronger.*)

CARO It really does feel like that, doesn't it?

JONATHAN Oh, yeah. It totally does! That's the *only* thing that's important to you at the time … is this illness.

CARO (*incidentally, to* JACK) The light's *very* bright in here.

JONATHAN (*squinting*) That's what I was just finking …

JACK Let's just wait.

(*The interview momentarily lapses whilst everyone waits for the extra-strong sunlight to subside.*)

CARO (*casually*) Sorry, Jon. We'll get up and running in a bit. (*Pause*) Yeah. I think that *is* kind of hard for young people. It's that idea that just when you're getting to that age when you're allowed to do more…

JONATHAN (*quickly*) Yeah! I was just getting to know myself and, yer know, just like *really* starting to take-off! *Really* starting to think about my exams. Starting to think about what I wanted to do when I was older, yer know, that type of fing. And all of a sudden it just … stops! And nothing else happens apart from hospital; feeling sick; home; injections … an' all that!

CARO And that's really what you felt most angry about is it? Everyone else gets on with their normal lives …

JONATHAN (*nodding enthusiastically*) I know I felt angry that no-one … (*Then to himself*) No. I'm not gonna say that.

CARO (*persuasively*) Yeah. Go on. (*Pause*) You were embarrassed then weren't you? Go on.

JONATHAN No.

CARO Why not? I think that's *really* important 'cos you now aren't and that's been a big change, Jon; hasn't it?

JONATHAN Alright. I'll say it then, yeah?

CARO (*convincingly*) I think you *should*. I think there are a lot of kids out there who are sitting there feeling embarrassed. They've got to know that you once were but you've learnt from that.

JONATHAN But I don't know what I was embarrassed of! It's *so* silly.

CARO What was your over-riding feeling then: your over-riding emotion?

JONATHAN I was embarrassed that people would come in and visit me and see me in such a state! I look back on it now: it couldn't be helped. But I don't know *why* I was embarrassed. I regret not letting people be close to me an' just being able to share fings with people. That's what I regret the most 'cos I was kind of embarrassed about what I looked like. How flushed I was. An' how horrible it was.

CARO What was the worst bit about the chemotherapy? Was it the physical thing, or was it the psychological kind of …? 'Cos it doesn't just affect you physically, does it? Does your head in a bit.

JONATHAN Yeah. It affects you mentally more than it does physically. Plays on yer mind constantly. I might be doing something else but it's always in the back of my head just reminding me. (JONATHAN *points to the back of his head.*)

CARO Is that because when you're thinking like that you're thinking: "Cancer. That's life-threatening. That might mean I die?"

JONATHAN (*calmly*) Yeah, definitely. (JONATHAN *looks directly into* CAROLINE's *eyes and speaks to her in an exceptionally honest and open manner.*) There was always that fear of it coming back anyway 'cos you see people that go out an' say, "Oh, I'm fine.

The treatment worked terrific!" And not long later they're back in 'cos they've found out that it's come back in their lungs or their chest which is, yer know, what's happened with me. (*Slightly bewildered*) But I always thought I'd be the lucky one. You always hear about this one odd person that goes home and the treatments done like really well and they get off an' running again. I always thought I'd be that person. I s'pose everyone does really 'cos they don't want to think that deep into it 'cos it's so hard.

CARO Can you explain, Jonathan? That was only about three or four weeks ago.

JONATHAN (*enthusiastically*) Yeah! I was like all clear. I had somefing in my lungs but that had all gone – supposedly! The problem in my foot had gone. And, erm, I was just so shocked because I've gone back for C.T. scans previously, yeah? (JONATHAN *mimics speech*) "Everything's fine, Jonathan. Now go home and live your life. Be an old man!" But, erm, about three or four weeks ago that wasn't to be. (*Pause*) I know it was three or four weeks ago but it seems like ages ago now. Seems like about six months ago.

(*Long pause*)

CARO What was your immediate thought?

JONATHAN Argh! I felt worse than when I was first diagnosed! *That* didn't feel half as bad to what I felt back in there 'cos I knew what my options would be. An' I knew how bad it would be whereas I didn't before. So I just couldn't believe it! Mum: she's gone out in tears. She went out of the room and Tori's gone after her and started talking to her an' I was sitting there for about fifteen minutes. I wasn't saying a word. I couldn't even think. I was going like this (JONATHAN *frowns and his facial expression becomes highly perplexed as he speaks very slowly and thoughtfully.*) I was looking out the window … I just couldn't believe it! And Julian was sitting there waiting for me to say somefing (*he sniffs*). Then my mum's come back in with Tori and they're all looking at me (JONATHAN *now speaks very softly*) an' I was like: "Oh, no! What do I say?"

CARO Did you cry?

JONATHAN (*emphatically*) No!

CARO (*disbelievingly*) You *didn't* cry?

JONATHAN (*truthfully*) Not there and then. No.

CARO Why not?

(*Pause*)

JONATHAN I don't s'pose it would have done any good …not for my mum's sake, anyway. (*Pause*) 'Cos she was already in a state. I know how *she* feels 'cos she shows her emotions a lot more than me. Erm, an' I thought, "Well, if I start bursting into tears now then what's that gonna do to her?" She wouldn't stop crying then, would she? She'd feel a lot worse. Then I'd feel bad about it 'cos she'd feel a lot worse.

(*Pause*)

CARO Did you ever think that was possible? I remember you said to me the night before that you had actually talked to your mum.

JONATHAN Yeah. The night before I went up for that scan to get those results I actually discussed it with my mum and I said, "If this problem comes back again I'm not having any treatment." But I only said that finking that I'd be fine. I didn't actually give it that much thought. I gave it thought that I'd made-up my mind that I wasn't gonna have any treatment but I didn't seriously consider that it would *actually* come back. But my decision didn't change when I realised that it *had* come back. So I'm not gonna have any treatment for it … (*slowly*) because there's no point.

(*Pause*)

CARO So you've decided, after being told that it has come back, to have nothing?

JONATHAN Yeah.

CARO Can you explain that, Jon?

JONATHAN Well, we went through it for quite a while. We were talking about possible options like chemotherapy; that's the first fing. (JONATHAN *looks directly into* CAROLINE'S *eyes again.*) I couldn't have the four again 'cos that was just *so* potent. That would be too much pressure on my heart. So he suggested one of those chemotherapies – Etoposide – and then, erm, he explained … the long an' the short of it was he said eventually the chemotherapy wouldn't save my life. It wouldn't keep the illness away. It may keep it at bay for a couple of months but it wouldn't keep me alive. (JONATHAN *adopts a highly perplexed facial expression along with a strong inquisitive tone to his speech.*) So then I pondered on it for a while, like saying to myself: "Well, what's the good in feeling *that* bad – with the chemotherapy - on top of how I'm feeling already and having to die anyway? (JONATHAN *raises his eyebrows as though he were asking the question directly to* CAROLINE *herself.*) I mean, I might as well 'go' feeling as best as I can and in the best shape as I can be. (*Pause*) That's what *I* thought. But I actually knew - as soon as he told me - what my decision was but I didn't wanna say it there and then. I wanted my mum to have a bit more time to get her head around it – and ev'ryone else – before I actually told mum.

(*Pause*)

CARO (*gently*) So what did you do that day? Did you go home and talk about it?

JONATHAN (*thoughtfully*) I was just in such a state I couldn't fink straight that day. But we eventually discussed it a couple of days later. An' then there was Tori saying – Julian's secretary – she was saying, (JONATHAN *mimics speech*) "Oh, there's no pressure. You make a decision whenever you want. You don't need to make an immediate decision." But I felt like I did 'cos, I mean, it's growing quickly! I felt like I *did* have to make a decision. (*Factually*) So, eventually, I told my mum that I wasn't gonna have any treatment and, er, she rang an' told Tori; and, er, here we are today.

(*Pause*)

CARO And was that kind of …umm. Did it seem very clear to you? Did you just think, "I *know* that's what I want to do?"

JONATHAN Well, to have more treatment would have been false hope for me and I don't need false hope. There's some people that need it. Parents that need it. Patients that need it 'cos they have nothing else. I'm not saying that that's a bad decision because it's not. I mean, they might not *know* its false hope at the time but later on they might realise that it *was* false hope. But you can't blame them for that 'cos, I mean, people that haven't been in this situation before, I mean, they can't judge if that's a bad decision or a good decision. I mean, you can only make that decision when you're *in* the moment. And that's how it was for me. But I believe it's the best decision that I could have made. (*Pause*) I believe (JONATHAN *nods*) …yeah, that it's the best decision.

CARO Did it feel a huge relief to actually make the decision?

JONATHAN Yeah, it did. (JONATHAN *sighs*) Although I knew it in my head I just wanted everyone else to know and not be finking,

(JONATHAN *mimics speech*) "What's he gonna *say*? What's gonna happen?" 'Cos it was entirely *my* decision. (*Pause*) If I couldn't have made the decision my mum would have made it for me. An' if she couldn't have made it then Julian would have made it for us: for me. That's how it was. I didn't *want* Julian to make it. Or mum. I wanted myself to make it so that I could feel happy with it an' then I couldn't blame anyone else for anyfing. Not that I would but I wouldn't want it on *their* shoulders.

CARO So did you feel like you wanted to go back to Julian and just check that there was no chance of …? Did you want to check that there wasn't any hope? Do you know what I mean? Did you go back and say to him "be straight"?

JONATHAN Erm, well, we went back a couple of days later with a clearer head an', erm, (JONATHAN's *young face has become slightly flushed as he begins to tire*) we had questions in mind; questions on paper and we were like: (JONATHAN *mimics speech*) "Be totally honest, Julian. Don't fool us!" (*He looks directly into* CAROLINE's *eyes*) 'Cos that's the only way you can be in a situation like this, innit? You can't make a proper decision without having the complete truth. So we said, "Please be honest and tell us. Just tell us!" And he did.

CARO And he just said there's no point?

JONATHAN Well, he didn't say there's no point. He didn't want it to seem as if there was no hope. But I remember him saying, (JONATHAN *mimics speech*) "Next time you come back for a scan – if you have chemotherapy – next time you come back the chances are that it's more likely that it would have done nuffing at all. That it wouldn't have helped. And it's less likely that it would have helped or stayed the same."

CARO Was it partly that you didn't want any more treatment because you hated chemotherapy?

JONATHAN (*emphatically*) Yeah! Well, people don't actually understand how *bad* it is. It's not like having the flu. Or having a cold, or a chest infection, or anyfing like that. It just brings you down *so* much! I wouldn't wish it on anyone – put it that way - not even my worst enemy. That's why it wouldn't be fair on myself to go through the chemotherapy again.

(*Pause*)

CARO Was it weird because when you go into hospital with something like cancer … You just had a slightly sore foot, didn't you? And is that why chemotherapy's quite bad because it's a treatment that makes you feel worse than what you went in with? Some treatments kind of make you feel better.

JONATHAN (*quickly*) Yeah, but it doesn't! You've gotta get worse before you can get better. An' in a lot of cases you get worse even though you *don't* get better. That's what it was like with me. Although in the back of my mind I always thought I'd get better an' I'd come home and … I'd live. But in the back of my mind there was always this fing saying to me that I might not. But I always tended to push that to the back of my head and just ignore it an' say that I would get on with my life. (*Pause*) But you can only deal with a problem like that when you're hit with it. But I found it *so* weird that I responded so brilliantly. It had gone in my chest. The problem in my foot had gone. I mean, the "all clear" should mean the "all clear" shouldn't it? I mean, I don't want to blame anyone 'cos you can't really. And I don't feel resentful towards anyone. I think I wasn't prepared for it an' maybe that was *my* fault. Maybe I should have tried to think about it an' actually considered that it might come back. But I didn't. (*Pause*) Perhaps me being not prepared for it *was* my fault … kinda.

CARO But in a way you say that you had that niggling thing. Can you tell me who put the niggle in there?

JONATHAN I s'pose seeing all the other patients come back an', yer know, be worse off than me. I s'pose seeing that put that little thing inside me. There are people that have come back after they've been given the all clear.

CARO I think that *is* one of the most difficult things. (CAROLINE *suddenly becomes distracted.*) Is this the dustcart going around? (*She turns to* JACK) Are you alright with that in? Sounds quite noisy. (*To* JONATHAN) But I think seeing other people is what …

MAX (*to* CAROLINE) Hang-on for a sec 'cos he's coming around.

(*The interview momentarily lapses whilst the din from the noisy dustcart becomes increasingly louder. Meanwhile, JONATHAN suddenly becomes self-conscious when he notices that JACK is surreptitiously taking some close-up body shots.*)

JONATHAN (*incidentally, to* CAROLINE) What do I look like? What's my hair like?

CARO You look good!

JONATHAN (*touching his hair*) Is it fluffy?

CARO No. You look good. It's funny 'cos your hair …

MAX (*to* JONATHAN) Did you lose *all* your hair?

JONATHAN (*to* MAX) Yeah. Ev'ry last strand! It was awful. I *hated* the way I looked. I wore a woollen hat constantly.

CARO (*to* JONATHAN) So, I do think I'm gonna ask you a bit more about that time … What *does* chemotherapy do to you? What's the gammit of it? What's the bits you hated about chemotherapy?

JONATHAN So many! But, erm, not being able to eat was one of 'em. And losing all that weight I lost. My face was all like … (JONATHAN *sucks his cheeks inwards*); I was all white; an' ev'ry time I even looked at food it just put me off eating forever. (*He becomes very facially expressive*) It really makes yer feel nauseous ev'ry time you look at some food when you're on it.

CARO And does it make you feel depressed? Or do you, kind of, have weird …? Some people have hallucinations.

JONATHAN Weird? (*Pause*) Ahh, yeah; that's hallucinations. I never had them. But I had anxiety attacks a couple of times.

CARO I mean, if someone offered you all that again and said that there is a hope it would cure you?

JONATHAN Well, if there's a hope then it's summink that's definitely gotta be considered an' my answer would probably be yeah. Yeah! Well, you've gotta if there's a hope. But from Julian there was, "It's not gonna save your life even if you *do* have treatment." So, I mean, I had to fink about that. And that was just 'no' really. You gotta understand, don't yer? It's a bit hard to go through all that. I mean, I know anyone that's been on chemotherapy like what I was would understand what I mean. But it's hard for people who haven't to understand.

(*Pause*)

CARO Do you think all that changed you?

JONATHAN (*thoughtfully*) Yeah. I *think* so. Well, physically I'm the same, like my face an' ev'ryfing. Apart from my hair. It's got a bit of a wave when it was always straight like that (JONATHAN *points to a much earlier school photograph of himself that is hanging on the wall.*) See that picture up there: look, lovely and straight! But now it's all curly. But inside: definitely I've changed. (*Pause*) I think I'm a bit … the word… I'm a bit more (JONATHAN *speaks this word slowly*) considerate – that's the word … considerate. I consider people's feelings an' what they must be finking. An' I try to be a bit more understanding as well … of how they must be feeling 'cos I know what feeling bad is all about. That's changed me like that.

CARO Do you feel more grown-up?

JONATHAN Oh, yeah. Definitely. Yeah. Absolutely.

CARO *How* do you feel?

JONATHAN Just my outlook on things an' the way I deal with things. And the way I evaluate problems in my head. I don't just brush them off now. I fink about them an' try to give it the best thought as possible. Gather-up all the information I've got of a problem an' then just try to make a best decision from it by weighing-up the pros and cons an' just … (JONATHAN *is becoming visibly tired now*) doing the best I can really.

CARO Because some people say that having cancer …

JACK (*quietly*) Sorry, Caroline, but I need to change tape.

JACK *replaces the used video tape in his camera and the interview between* JONATHAN *and* CAROLINE *recommences from where it left off. All five characters are positioned as before. And the strong, mid-morning sun is still shining brightly through the big bay-window. It continues to highlight the entire right-hand side of* JONATHAN'*s handsome, young face giving him a soft, ethereal glow throughout.* (VICKI *speaks to camera*):

I FELT ACUTELY TENSE AND uneasy in the days leading

up to Jonathan's test results. Naturally, I gave much thought to the mysterious lump inside his left foot and constantly wondered what it could possibly be. My frazzled nerves were all over the place. In fact, to my shame, I went uncharacteristically berserk at Rosie one evening when she naively suggested that Jonathan "might have cancer":

"That's a *really horrible* fing to say!" I screeched at her. "Go to your room right now! And don't *ever* mention that *disgusting* word inside our house again. Not EVER!"

In floods of tears, Rosie dashed out of the front-room. Whilst Richard, Jonathan and Daniel sat perfectly silent.

However, later that same evening - when all the children were sleeping – I remained awake for a long time sobbing with worry and remorse. I eventually drifted into an exhausted sleep. But not before I had pleaded with God to keep my cherished son safe and well taking great care, of course, not to mention - let alone think about - that disgusting word Rosie had dared to mention much earlier -

JONATHAN (*to* MAX, *smiling*) I think that microphone's great. I want one!

MAX They're pricey.

JONATHAN How much are they?

MAX There's about two and a half grands worth in there.

JONATHAN (*smiling, whilst gently tapping* MAX's *microphone*) Does that hurt your ears?

(*A light sprinkling of dust falls on* JONATHAN's *head.*)

CARO (*suddenly, and professionally, to* JONATHAN) So, can you explain Jonathan – Is it a bit like on the one hand you feel like a kid again and on the one hand you feel like you're a lot wiser than everyone else?

JONATHAN (*flippantly*) Have I gotta say it in a sentence?

CARO No. I mean; *is* that true? Does it feel like …?

JONATHAN (*quickly*) Yeah. It *is* true. In some ways I feel like I'm growing-up 'cos of my thoughts and what I'm finking – as I've explained earlier – but in some ways I feel like I'm a baby again 'cos I need my mum so much. I rely on her for ev'ryfing.

CARO And that's hard 'cos all your friends are kind of growing-up and doing all the things that teenagers do and …

JONATHAN Yeah. And I've only just started to, yer know, like going out an' all that business. I was only starting to do it an', I mean, got cut-off from ev'ryone; from all the crowd. Whilst they carried on I was in slow-motion. Not progressing one bit.

CARO And in the time that you were given the all clear and you were back at home were you able to be normal?

JONATHAN Yeah. That was great! That was a good time. I'm grateful for that time 'cos a lot of people don't have that. A lot of people don't get better. They go into hospital ill an' they don't come out of hospital. But I try and look at it as being fortunate that I had the time - after being ill - I had the time to go home an' live again. Yer know, just do the general stuff that people do. I had about six months, or summink, to get back to school; meet my friends; go out; enjoy being with the family – an' all that. I had just a bit extra whereas a lot of people don't have that so I was grateful for that really.

CARO And when you were told that it had come back, Jonathan, and you thought, "I'm not going to have the treatment": what have you decided? If you're not going into hospital how are you gonna spend the next few weeks and months? What do you feel is … ? (*Pause*) Why *not* have treatment?

JONATHAN (*slowly*) Because it's not going to work how I want it to work an' then keep me alive. I mean, my life might be a bit longer but just that fraction bit longer. And what's that bit of life worth when you're feeling like death warmed up? (*Pause*) It's not … well, in my mind, it's not worth it. That's only in my mind anyway. That's only how I see it.

(*Pause*)

CARO So what do you want to do? Like go to Disneyland, or …?

JONATHAN (*adamantly*) Na! Don't be silly! I haven't got a list like all that. (JONATHAN *mimics hurried speech*) "Gotta do this, blah blah blah!" I don't do that. I don't *wanna* do that! I just like being at home an' just living normal. Not skitting off to Disneyland and meeting people. Not that. No. I just wanna be at home and just be as I was before, really. And see, obviously, maybe that bit more of people that are special to me … Anyway, I'm going to Lourdes tomorrow so that's summink.

CARO And do you find that now, having sort of, now there's nothing anyone can do to cure it ... Do you feel like you're having to confront the whole idea of death?

JONATHAN Yeah.

CARO Do you think about it a lot?

JONATHAN Well, yeah. It's in my mind constantly. I've said before: it's in my mind.

CARO What is?

JONATHAN Always playing on me. The idea that it's gonna happen.

CARO But now what's …? The idea that …

JONATHAN *When* it's gonna happen! *That's* what's playing on my mind. The idea it's gonna … one day. Maybe not suddenly but … still: it's still summink to think about, innit? Maybe I don't wanna think about it but I got to! Forced to. Can't get out of it.

CARO I mean, most people are really scared to think about it like that. Are *you* scared?

JONATHAN No. I'm not scared. Not for me anyway. (*Defensively*) I don't wanna seem like someone who's like really big and, yer know, (JONATHAN *mimics speech*) "*I'm* not scared!" But I'm more scared for my family and how they're gonna cope 'cos they've gotta live with that, ain't they? They've gotta live with what's happened an' I don't!

CARO And it must feel weird 'cos at the moment do you *feel* like there's anything wrong with you?

JONATHAN No.

JONATHAN I've said it before. It's so weird 'cos I know inside I'm not physically okay. I know there's a lot wrong but I haven't felt *this* good in myself as I have in two years. I feel great physically. I don't feel like there's nuffing wrong with me.

CARO So do you find it hard to believe?

JONATHAN I *believe* it but it's hard to take in. It's hard to suss it all out 'cos (JONATHAN *mimics speech*) "Hang-on. Why am I feeling so good if I'm *not* good!?"

CARO And do you find that every day you're waiting to see when it's going to … when you're going to start feeling …?

JONATHAN (*nodding*) Mmm, I'm waiting. (*Pause*) I'm just waiting for the breathlessness to start 'cos I know that's one of the first fings. You start getting out of breath an' you have to have the oxygen. But it's always different for ev'ryone: the timing.

CARO Do you *want* to know?

JONATHAN (*honestly*) Yeah. I *would* like to know how long I've got and when it's gonna happen 'cos then I've got more information inside my head. And then I can plan fings and … (*pause*) I've got a bit more perspective of what's gonna happen. Got more reality. D'yer know what I mean? (*Nodding*) Yeah. I'd rather know.

(*Pause*)

CARO Do you have any idea at the moment? Does it *feel* like you know? 'Cos you're usually quite clear about …

JONATHAN (*sighs heavily*) I don't. (*Pause*) (JONATHAN *chooses his words very carefully before he continues.*) I've got ideas. But they may not be right 'cos I've never been through it before. (*Reluctantly shaking his head*) I'm not gonna say. I'm not gonna have a guess 'cos that's just silly, innit? Guessing before you know how long I've got left, that's not a very wise thing to do. (*Openly*) 'Cos I *don't* know really, do I?

CARO So, what? Are you gonna go to the clinic to ask them?

JONATHAN Yeah. See what he's gotta say for himself: Julian. See if he can give me any more new information.

CARO What do you want to know from him?

JONATHAN Well, whatever *they* know I wanna know. (JONATHAN *sighs*) Whatever they've gotta tell me then I just wanna know ev'ryfing, really. (JONATHAN *looks directly into* CAROLINE's *eyes*)

I'm not scared of knowing.

(*Pause*)

CARO 'Cos I think some people *are* really scared and that's why …
(*Quickly*) Where *do* you get that kind of …Why *aren't* you scared,
Jonathan?

JONATHAN (*grinning widely at* CAROLINE) Why *aren't* I scared?
(JONATHAN *considers his words very carefully*) I s'pose it's got a lot
to do with my faith and my religion: what I believe in. It gives me a bit
more inner-strength an' inner-peace with myself.

CARO Have you always been religious?

JONATHAN (*brightly*) Yeah!

(*Nervously,* JONATHAN *fiddles with his gold cross pendant that has
been loosely hanging outside his jumper throughout. He carefully
straightens the chain and puts the cross inside his jumper before
quickly pulling it back out again.*)

CARO Can you explain that to me? I mean, it's not just something
you've suddenly gone …

JONATHAN (*defensively*) No! I haven't just suddenly '*gone*'.
Although there's nuffing wrong with that I s'pose. But I've always
gone to church. Ever since I was small I've always gone to church
ev'ry Sunday an' all that. Altar serving. I've always believed in God
and it's not just something that's just turned about now: it's something
that's always been a part of me. But summink like this brings it out in
me more. Just *this.* This predicament and what's going on.

CARO Did it help you last year when you …?

JONATHAN (*enthusiastically*) Oh, yeah! I mean, when someone that

doesn't have any faith in anything – and they're in a problem like me
- a lot of them would just turn to cracking-up. They'd turn to alcohol;
drugs, yer know, over-dosing. All that. But I didn't. I didn't turn to
anything like that: cracking-up or anyfing. I just turned to my faith and
my beliefs an' I believe I got inner-peace from it and just a bit more
inner-strength to be able to deal with what's going on and what's gonna
happen in the future.

CARO Did you pray to God to make you better?
JONATHAN (*truthfully*) Yeah, well … I mean: I can't question God's
will can I? Whatever He's got in plan then I can't … If He wants to
make me better then He would. If He doesn't then He won't.

(*Pause*)

CARO So when you found out it came back you didn't feel angry with
God?

JONATHAN (*quickly*) No. Not at all.

CARO How? Can you explain? Is that because you believe?

JONATHAN (*quickly*) Yeah! I mean, I don't believe that life stops
here on this earth. I believe that I'll go into another life and just have
a lot more important things to do than what's going on down here.
There's a lot more important stuff going on, I believe, anyway. And I
fink I'll have a part of that. (*Resignedly*) That's why I'm not angry …
or scared, really. That's why I'm not that scared 'cos I believe in that.

(*Pause*)

CARO *What* do you believe? Can you explain what your vision of
things after earth is?

(JONATHAN *thinks long and carefully before he eventually responds
to the question.*)

JONATHAN (*shaking his head*) Not gonna. Can't.

CARO You can't?

JONATHAN No. 'Cos …

CARO Maybe you could just explain to me you can't really explain it because it's private, or it's something …

JONATHAN Yeah. I fink ev'ryone's got their own idea of what the afterlife is an' for me to say what mine is might ruin someone else's perception so I fink it's best left inside of me and let everyone else have their own ideas of what it's like so I won't disappoint anyone, or make 'em – yer know?

(*Pause*)

CARO But do you *really* feel like you know what …?

JONATHAN (*playfully*) Huh?

CARO But you *really* feel like you do …? But I'm just … I think it's helpful to people when you have a kind of faith like you have, Jonathan. It's like you don't have to feel so scared, do you? 'Cos …

JONATHAN 'Cos it's not it! Yeah!

CARO You have a clear sight.

(*Together*)

JONATHAN (*enthusiastically*) Yeah!

CARO Can you explain?

JONATHAN What, have a clear sight? Well, yeah: I s'pose that *is* why I'm not scared 'cos I have a clear sight of what's gonna happen an' I don't just think that I've had this illness and I'm coming along the line an' finally it stops there. I don't think there's a barrier there. I think I'll go straight on an' just pass it all. Leave it all behind and just move on. That's why I've got a clear head and just try an' fink straightforward. And don't get all muddled.

CARO You know, we talked earlier, didn't we? When you were asked, "What do you want to do?" You just *knew*, didn't you?

JONATHAN Yeah!

CARO Is it something that God comes …

JONATHAN (*very quietly*) Yeah.

CARO God tells you …

(*Together*)

JONATHAN (*very quietly*) Although I didn't say it …

CARO *Did* God help you make those decisions?

JONATHAN Probably. Yeah. Ahh, I don't know. (*Then bluntly*) It would have happened anyway. I would … I would … die anyway, so … there's a lot I don't understand anyway so I can't really, yer know, say a lot about it. I don't really understand that much of what's going on elsewhere so I'm not gonna go an' say.

CARO (*relentlessly*) But it's almost like your faith, isn't it?

JONATHAN Yeah, that's what it is. That's faith.

CARO Your faith means it doesn't matter if you don't have all the answers. Is that right?

JONATHAN Mmm, yeah.

CARO Do you know what I mean? Is that right?

JONATHAN Mmm, yeah. You've got it in one.

CARO Can you explain that?

JONATHAN *Can* I explain it? Erm …

CARO (*quickly*) Well, it's almost like … People are gonna say, "How come you have such strength and you *are not* scared, Jonathan?" 'Cos I really believe you're *not* scared. I'm sure there are times when you have some fear. And you feel a bit frightened, obviously. But I think I know you well enough now to say that, you know; you really *aren't* terrified.

JONATHAN (*shakes his head in agreement*) Ah, ah …

CARO (*Quickly*) And I just think for people to understand where that comes from. It's not a cockiness. It's not …

JONATHAN (*very defensively*) It's *not* a cockiness! I don't want it to seem as if it's cockiness.

CARO (*quickly*) No. No. No. I'm not saying it is but that's why I'm trying to … I'm not trying to get you to say things that are very personal to you but try to think of ways to express to people that, you know, it's just about having a kind of faith, isn't it?

(*Pause*)

JONATHAN How shall I put it then?

CARO (*casually*) I don't know. *Don't* put it if you don't … (*She clears her throat*) I just think it's *really* interesting.

JONATHAN (*courageously*) Alright then.

CARO (*quickly*) I mean, for a start, you've had spiritual experiences that have given you that kind of … You *feel* like you know.

JONATHAN (*half smiling*) Yeah. I told you about that, didn't I?

CARO Yeah. I mean, you don't have to describe them …

(*Together*)

JONATHAN (*very quietly, more to himself*) Not *all* about them …

CARO (*relentlessly*) But you *have*, haven't you?

JONATHAN (*decisively and firmly*) I'm not gonna go into that. I'll leave that with myself.

CARO You don't want to even mention that you've had …? There are things that have happened to you that have …?

(*Pause*)

Well, I think it's really special, Jon.

JONATHAN (*faltering*) Yeah, but … it's *personal*. It's a bit …

CARO (*softly*) Yeah … But you don't have to describe …

(*Together*)

JONATHAN (*pleadingly*) No-one else will understand!

CARO No. And I'm not trying …

JONATHAN (*quietly*) No-one else would understand it really …

(*Together*)

CARO If you've obviously …

A lot of people who find faith difficult will find it … (CAROLINE *is suddenly distracted by a very loud bang that has come from inside the kitchen.*) (*Agitated, she calls out to* JACK) You alright?

JONATHAN (*cheerily*) He's looking at the tele in there.

CARO Mmm … You know, who find it hard to have faith because they feel they have no proof, don't they? But in a way, *your* faith has given you a real sense of belief.

(JONATHAN *reaches for his bottle of natural spring water. He opens the lid and takes a small drink of water before quietly agreeing with* CAROLINE. *He half smiles at her; sighs heavily; and then softly mumbles to himself as he struggles to find the correct words that will best express how he is feeling towards her relentless questioning.*)

JONATHAN (*coyly*) I don't know how to put. (*Long pause.* JONATHAN *looks directly into the camera.*) Is it still going on?

CARO (*quickly and casually*) Mmm …

JONATHAN (*submissively*) Well, how do you want me to say it then?

CARO (*quickly*) You say it how you wanna say it - if you think it's important. How do you think it will help people to understand what you … where you get your strength from?

(*Pause*)

JONATHAN (*boldly*) Well, it's just faith! That's it! I can't … (*Long pause.* JONATHAN *now speaks hesitantly but very precisely.*) There's doubt in people's minds that things … don't go on … but I don't have a doubt, really. And I've …had proof that there's no … that … there's … (*quickly*) a life after death. I've had proof. But that's personal to me and I won't go into it. So, I don't know, it's just … I don't know how to tell other people to deal with it, or … (*directly to* CAROLINE) You can't tell someone else to get faith, can you? It's gotta come from them, so … (JONATHAN *instinctively reaches for his gold cross pendant and lightly taps his chest with it.*)

(*Pause*)

CARO Do you feel lucky, though, that you've had that faith to help you?

JONATHAN Oh, yeah! If I didn't have the faith I wouldn't have nuffing. I would have crumbled! Honestly, I would have. That's what kept me together really.

(*Long pause.* JONATHAN, *appearing slightly uncomfortably, once again feels for his gold cross pendant. He then softly nods at* CAROLINE *in a highly perceptive and insightful way.*)

CARO (*professionally*) And is that why, in the next few weeks, you want to … Things like Lourdes … But some people will say, "So why aren't you going to Disneyland and mucking around and …"

JONATHAN (*quickly, and half smiling*) 'Cos I don't like Disneyland!

CARO (*lightly*) *Do* people say that to you? Can you explain that to me? *Have* people said that?

JONATHAN Well, I've had a couple of people say (JONATHAN *speaks quickly as he mimics speech.*) "Oh, you should really be doing stuff now. You should be going here; you should be going there." (*Determinedly*) But *they* can't tell me what to do! They don't know how it feels! I've gotta do what I want, really, without trying to sound arrogant. I've gotta keep *myself* happy an' just do what I feel would help me the most and be best for me. And I think skitting off to Disneyland an' all that, which is what people tend to do, I don't fink would be within my interests. (JONATHAN *shrugs*) So there you go!

CARO And there are things that you want to do that bring you closer to God? Would *that* be right? Are there things that you want to do that make you … Is going to see the Pope, and Lourdes, are they …?

JONATHAN Oh, yeah; seeing the Pope. Yeah. Well, that was actually arranged without me knowing.

JACK (*coughs lightly*) Caroline! I'm *really* struggling on the light now.

CARO Are you? OK. Let's just cut!

JACK *replaces the used video tape in his camera and the interview between* JONATHAN *and* CAROLINE *recommences from where it left off. All five characters are positioned as before. The strong, mid-morning sun is still shining brightly through the big bay-window. It continues to highlight the entire right-hand side of* JONATHAN'*s handsome, young face giving him a soft, ethereal glow throughout.* (VICKI *speaks to camera*):

I SOON BECAME AN EXPERT at hiding my anxiety from the children. Indeed, for their sake, I did my utmost to appear happy and normal. And yet, hard as I tried, nothing could prevent me from trembling each time the telephone rang. Thankfully, Doctor Raj contacted us just three days after Jonathan's hurried tests and luckily the children were still at school:

"Is that Mrs James?" He asked, professionally.

"It is." I quickly told him.

"Hello. This is Doctor Raj from the Greenwich District Hospital." There was a long silence. "Erm, I'm ringing to inform you about Jonathan's test results." There was another long silence. "Mrs James?" He enquired.

"Yes." I eventually whispered.

"It appears Jonathan *does* have a tumour in his foot but he will need further tests before we can ascertain whether it is malignant or …"

"*Malignant!*" I rudely interrupted.

"I'm not saying …" continued the careful doctor.

"Then what *are* you saying?" I interrupted again.

"I'm saying that Jonathan will need further tests. Doctor Patel has referred your son to The Royal National Orthopaedic Hospital in Stanmore." There was another long silence. "You should hear from them …"

"A *tumour*?" I cried.

"Yes." He simply told me.

"But how … I mean, what … *How* will you cure him?" I desperately asked.

"That will be down to Stanmore. You should hear from them very soon." He concluded.

"But it's the Millennium, Doctor! Oh my God! It's gonna be a *long* Christmas!" -

CARO (*professional, yet friendly*) So, Jonathan: how you gonna cope with the next few weeks? (*Quickly*) What do you see happening? You say you're waiting until …

JONATHAN (*quickly*) I'm gonna take every day as it comes. I'm just gonna live for today an' do what I want *today*. Tomorrow: maybe do summink different. Just take things one step at a time. I'm not gonna plan ahead or anyfing.

CARO (*quickly*) Is it weird thinking: "I'm not gonna live?"

JONATHAN Yeah. It was weird in school the other week because I was in there an' I was doing what I normally do: going to the lessons; listening an' all that. And then he started handing out the exam papers. And they're all talking about their mock exams; their real exams; what they wanna do; what they wanna achieve. And I'm sitting there an' even though they might not all be looking at me that's what I feel like because I feel like they're all finking, (JONATHAN *mimics speech*) "What's *he* thinking 'cos he ain't gonna have to do this!" And, like, they're all working towards their futures *now* and I'm … not.

(*Pause*)

CARO (*quickly*) It's quite *hard* to know how to live knowing that you don't have a future, isn't it?

JONATHAN Yeah.

CARO 'Cos in a way we're all conditioned.

JONATHAN Yeah! Ev'ryone's conditioned to work towards summink they like an' what they wanna be and that's what everyone's doing at the moment. And I'm finking (JONATHAN *mimics speech*) "Damn! This is strange! I haven't got a goal!" It's weird. Very weird.

CARO Before all this happened, did you think to yourself, "Oh, when I'm thirty I'll have kids and I'll be doing …?"

JONATHAN Yeah.

CARO *How* did you see yourself?

JONATHAN Well, I think everyone does, don't they? Everyone thinks the best for themselves and wants to achieve the best that they can do. (*Factually*) Like marry at thirty; have a couple of kids – boy an' a girl – yer know: that silly stuff. Nice job; nice house; nice garage (JONATHAN *draws an illusory garage with his finger*). All that. (*Pause*) But it's not how it works out sometimes, is it? That's not reality.

CARO Is that how you saw life panning out for yourself?

JONATHAN Yeah. I fink everyone does. I mean, it's only natural, isn't it? To look ahead and to want the best for yourself and to have a family an' want the best for them. But in reality that's not how it is, is it? Reality is some people get there and some people don't. Some people are taken at …Some people die at one week old; some people die a hundred years old. It's different for ev'ryone. (*Pause*) But no-one expects this. Ev'ryone just expects the best, really. So did I.

(*Pause*)

CARO (*gently*) And when you say you don't really have a goal anymore is your goal, in a way, making sure you have the best time. I mean, what *is* your goal then?

JONATHAN It's … Ohh … (JONATHAN *sighs heavily; frowns; and then looks downwards in an attempt to find the correct words that will sufficiently answer* CAROLINE'*s difficult question.*) (*To himself*) How can I put it? (*Pause*) Just being on good terms with ev'ryone.

CARO I mean, do you feel like you're preparing … to die, Jon?

JONATHAN (*softly*) Yeah.

CARO (*lightly*) Is that what it feels like?

JONATHAN Yeah. Preparing. It *does* feel like that.

CARO Can you explain *that* to me?

JONATHAN Yeah. I wanna get ev'ryone on my side. Before, there was people with me, yer know, *like* me – and then there was people over there that perhaps I didn't make an effort with, or didn't make an effort with me. And I wanna, yer know, get everyone on my side and just get along with ev'ryone now, I suppose. So I can part on good terms.

CARO And have you thought about the *way* you want to die and *how* you want to die?

JONATHAN (*quickly*) Home! In bed!

CARO Can you explain that? You and your mum have talked about it, have you?

JONATHAN (*looking towards the floor, he sighs heavily and toys with his gold cross pendant as he speaks.*) Well, the decision *not* to have chemotherapy …what comes wiv that is being able to live here and die here. I mean, that comes wiv it. 'Cos if I have chemotherapy then I'd be in hospital; perhaps maybe die in hospital. But not having chemotherapy: I'll 'go' here. (*Slowly*) And I think that's felt with my mum as well. (JONATHAN *looks towards the ceiling and points to the exact spot where his bed is situated upstairs. He continues to speak in a casual and open manner.*) Upstairs in my room. Up there. Just … as normal.

(*Long pause*)

CARO And you'll take pain-killers and whatever else they …?

JONATHAN Well, whatever. (*Resignedly*) Whatever life throws at me in the future – pain wise – I'm sure that I'll be able to side-step the pain with some pills or any type of drugs, or whatever they've got. I'm sure they'll do their best to keep the pain at bay for me.

CARO Does the physical side of it not really worry you?

JONATHAN (*tiredly*) I haven't really thought about it. I've been finking about the ultimate … ending. I haven't been finking about the consequences leading up to it that much.

CARO And *that's* your way of dealing with it, isn't it?

JONATHAN (*quickly*) Just take it as it comes! I mean, there's no point of planning ahead – that's not gonna get me nowhere. No point of finking about (JONATHAN *mimics speech*) "Oh, am I gonna feel *this* pain; am I gonna feel *that* pain." I mean, if I worry about that then I can't live now, can I? An' I wanna just do the best I can to live now.

CARO What about the pain in your shoulder?

JONATHAN (*sighs*) Yeah, well … (*he slips his right hand into the top of his jumper and lightly pats his left shoulder.*) I've had it there for a couple of weeks. (JONATHAN *softly rubs his left shoulder*) I'm still unsure what it is but … (*He looks at* CAROLINE *in a very insightful manner*) yer know, there's an inclination of what it probably is.

CARO What was your immediate reaction? That I want some treatment?

JONATHAN (*still toying with his gold cross pendant*) No. (*Then quickly*) That hasn't changed! That thought hasn't changed about wanting treatment. I still don't want treatment. (*Pause.* JONATHAN *touches his left shoulder again*) I s'pose this all comes with it, doesn't it? The choice of not having treatment – all this business you gotta deal wiv. (*Softly*) That's just part and parcel.

CARO Who's been your main support?

JONATHAN (*Quickly*) My mum!

CARO Can you explain that to me?

JONATHAN Yeah. Well, ev'ry time I've gone to a hospital appointment she's been there wiv me. She's been asking questions. She's been taking the questions home an' talking about them wiv me. Ev'ry round of treatment I've had she's been there: day and night. She's slept over there a couple of times in hospital 'cos she didn't wanna leave. Ev'ryfing. Every problem that we've encountered I say 'we' 'cos she's dealt with it with me. She's had to carry as much as I've had to carry really.

CARO Do you think it's as hard for the mums?

JONATHAN I think it's *harder* for the mums! I really do fink it's harder. Just as hard, at least! Definitely hard for my mum. Well, at least *just* as hard because they're feeling ev'ryfing that their child is feeling. They're there with them all the time and they're gonna have to live wiv it after the consequences have happened. They're gonna have to live with those consequences. And maybe even blame themselves even though they shouldn't. They're gonna have to live with all that, ain't they? It's summink that's gonna be with them forever.

CARO Have you two always been close?

JONATHAN Oh, yeah. My mum and I have always been close ever since I was tiny. We've always had this special bond together an' this has brought that special bond … just brought us that bit closer. And we understand each other a bit more, although we always did anyway. But this just made it that more … *special* between us.

CARO Do you share your faith as well?

JONATHAN (*brightly*) Yeah!

CARO It's not just that you're quite similar as people.

JONATHAN We *are* quite similar as people. But, yeah, we share our faith. I mean, she's the one who gave me my faith when I was little. When I was little she was the one who brought me to church and taught me this, taught me that an', yeah, she's the one that shares all that wiv me. I can tell her anyfing, really. Nuffing she doesn't know anyway that I don't know. I fink we know both the same.

CARO Do you come from a very strong …?

JACK (*quietly*) Erm, sorry Caroline, but we've almost reached the end of the tape.

(VICKI *speaks to camera*):

INITIALLY, I DECIDED TO PROLONG telling Jonathan about my conversation with Doctor Raj because I wanted to protect him from the worry for as long as possible. However, my plan soon changed when, by four-thirty that same afternoon, Jonathan and Daniel refused to stop wrestling together inside our tiny front-room.

"For *God's* sake, Jonathan! You *have* to listen to me!" I pleaded from inside the kitchen doorway. He still ignored me. So I hurriedly continued: "The hospital rang today. They said you've got a tumour inside yer foot!"

The boy's wrestling bout abruptly ended. Jonathan's flushed face peered up at me from the floor. He looked puzzled.

"But I feel okay, Mum: not ill or nuffing." He panted.

"I know, babes." I softly sympathized. " But you *can't* knock yer foot just in case …" I almost cried.

Jonathan dragged himself onto the shabby-pink sofa. Daniel and I joined him. And, together, we discussed my recent conversation with Doctor Raj.

"But how will they remove the lump wivout damaging my foot?" Jonathan asked.

"Can't say right now, babes. All we can do is wait an' see." I told him.

"Well, let's hope it don't take too long to sort out 'cos I've got a busy year ahead, what wiv my exams an' ev'ryfing!" Jonathan logically stated.

Daniel and I wholeheartedly agreed. But, needless to say, our final Christmas in the twentieth century was not filled with great joy and anticipation for the approaching New Millennium. Instead, it was filled with much worry and concern for Jonathan's health. Thankfully, our appointment at Stanmore Hospital arrived within just seven days. Nevertheless, in truth, it was the longest week I had ever known. Yet, somehow, I held it all together with the happy and familiar sounds of Elvis Costello, Madonna and Cher; tackling lots of household chores; whilst drinking plenty of delicious French and Italian white wine! In fact, surprisingly, I arrived at Stanmore feeling utterly convinced that Jonathan's tumour was most definitely; no doubt about it; one hundred percent benign. It simply *had* to be.

At the same time, I awoke extra-early one morning to discover an old photograph of our long-deceased Grandma Rose sitting on top of the dining table. I was more than astonished and perplexed because I felt certain that it was not there the night before. Regardless, a warm tear rolled down my cheek as I fondly stared into Grandma's wise old face. But I soon smiled again when I recollected the day she visited me at the Greenwich District Hospital just hours after Jonathan's late delivery. She was *so* excited to meet him. And here she was again, smiling back at me with my serene son cradled in her loving arms on that hot and humid Sunday in mid-August, 1985.

"Have you been down my old suitcase?" I routinely asked each child, as they awoke that same morning. But they all emphatically denied having anything to do with the photograph's mysterious appearance. And because I knew that it could only have come from one place, I immediately dashed upstairs and searched through Rosie's in-built wardrobe. However, once again, I was totally amazed to discover that my old suitcase had, indeed, been untouched by their prying little hands! Anyhow, because it was such a lovely photograph of Grandma, I soon found a suitable frame and proudly displayed it on my bedside cabinet. Exactly one week later, Jonathan was finally diagnosed with a Synovial Sarcoma inside his left foot. And our whole family life was instantly turned upside down.

Scene closes to 'The Sound of Silence'
sung by Simon and Garfunkel.

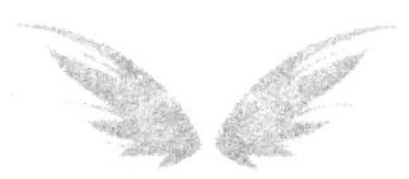

ACT TWO

Let It Be

Introducing

DOCTOR JULIAN, a leading London Oncologist. Tall and lean; extra-large, dark-brown eyes; and short, mid-brown hair. Courteous; considerate; and mild-mannered. An expert in his field, he is exceptionally well-groomed and professional at all times. His highly-educated, British accent lacks any hint of superiority.

TORI, a Clinical Nurse Specialist for teenagers with cancer. Average height; mildly plump; soft-hazel eyes; and short, light-brown hair that is noticeably lighter at the crown and fringe. Extremely friendly; warm-natured; and compassionate. She frequently smiles as she speaks in her fast-paced, London accent.

Setting: An Oncology Clinic in a busy central London Hospital.

SCENE ONE

19th February, 2001: *It is mid-morning. The Oncology Clinic is pleasantly decorated with cream coloured walls; lemon flooring; and light, beech-wood furnishings. And* JONATHAN (*wearing a thin, black jumper; light-blue trousers; and a black, woollen jacket*) *along with* VICKI (*wearing a navy, fleece cardigan; beige trousers; and blue denim jacket*) *have arrived early for their appointment to see* DOCTOR JULIAN. *They are seated in the middle of a long line of brown-padded chairs, opposite reception where* JACK *has set-up a running camera. A large cylinder of water – with plastic cups - is situated to their right. Presently, a team of young doctors gather around the reception desk. With clenched fists stuffed inside the pockets of their white, shapeless overcoats they peruse the medical files that are neatly arranged on top of the wide counter. Meanwhile,* VICKI, *lost inside her own private thoughts, is observing* JONATHAN's *left knee that is bouncing up and down in its usual rapid manner. But when he suddenly spots his mother's lost and vacant stare, she averts her tired gaze towards the heavy double -doors that lead into the clinic, which is still quite empty.* (*She speaks to camera*):

I AWOKE EARLIER THAN USUAL this morning amid a vivid dream in which I was driving in slow motion down a vast, concrete motorway. Huge, grey blocks engulfed me. The wide road seemed never-ending. Indeed, the fear I felt at being so lost and alone in such a hectic and unfamiliar place stayed with me even after waking. Staring at the mottled ceiling inside my tiny box-room, my racing heart thumped loudly. I struggled to calm my breathing. Desperate, I sought solace in the lingering memory I had of a kind- looking, elderly gentleman whose friendly face periodically smiled at me through my nearside window. But still my anxious thoughts returned to the hordes of faceless drivers who recklessly zipped past me like wild, uncontrollable junkies from a crazy road-trip movie. It was *such* a relief to wake-up and discover it was only a dream because it felt as though my whole life depended on which lane I was about to choose. Anyhow, safe inside the inky darkness of my cosy bedroom, I soon became distracted by Jonathan's dry, persistent cough that has steadily worsened over the past few days. Gradually, his harsh, hacking bark permeated the whole house. And I thought it amazing how the children could sleep through such a loud, discordant noise including Jonathan himself! I attempted to pray. But the only words I heard inside my muddled mind was Caroline's trained voice, repeatedly asking: *Do you ever feel angry with God because Jonathan got cancer*? Closely followed by my own nonchalant reply, echoing: *Na, 'course not! Diseases ain't caused by God so why blame Him for ev'ryfing*? But that was easier to say in January. Jonathan's symptoms have changed a lot since then. And so have I –

JONATHAN (*to* VICKI, *sighing and leaning forward in his seat.*) D'ya reckon Caroline's already in there? It's gonna be well cramped. (VICKI*'s heavy eyes survey her cherished son's dampened hair that has been meticulously styled to appear natural yet smart. She smiles at him: a warm, affectionate smile to which he instantly responds. Her loving gaze lingers over his extremely pale complexion. She blinks away an unexpected tear before she is thankfully distracted by* JONATHAN*'s gold cross pendant that is glistening beneath the clinic's halogen lamps.*) D'ya fink they'll be long? I'm popping to the loo quickly! (*Still silent,* VICKI *taps* JONATHAN*'s left arm before he rises from his seat; dashes past reception; and then disappears through some big beech-wood doors. She speaks to camera*):

SADLY, MY FRETFUL MIND FAILED to ease with the fading darkness. Instead, powerful feelings of guilt, remorse and especially pity for Jonathan gradually overwhelmed me. Alone in those early hours – before the children awoke - I could do no more than weep at the sheer hopelessness of our situation, along with the stark realisation of knowing that my fierce maternal instincts now count for nothing against our invisible enemy who has, in truth, long beaten us. But the harsh reality of having no choice other than to accept Jonathan's untimely death and to witness his personal suffering is crucifying me too. So now I don't trust in God anymore. I believe He has let us all down. And I'm certain Richard, Daniel and Rosie feel this way too. And yet, despite his dire circumstances Jonathan's Christian faith is growing stronger by the day. He prays a lot. And whenever he tells me about the amazing spiritual experiences he still receives, it is comforting to know that at least *he* feels loved by God which is some consolation to me at this time. Anyhow, we all attended the mass together yesterday evening. And although I now go mostly out of habit, I admit there is a tiny part of me that still believes it is the right thing to do -

JONATHAN *returns to his seat beside* VICKI. *Then, within seconds,* TORI (*wearing a baggy, bottle-green shirt; black jumper; and black trousers*) *appears at the far end of the waiting area. Her soft-round face reveals few signs of make-up but for a dash of brown eye-shadow; a touch of mascara; and a lick of light-pink lipstick. Realising that she has been spotted,* TORI *smiles at* JONATHAN *and* VICKI *before scurrying down the small wooden staircase to greet them. The trio exchange some brief pleasantries together before* TORI *leads* JONATHAN *and* VICKI *back up the staircase. They linger on the crescent-shaped landing where several big beech-wood doors - all firmly closed - surround them. Presently,* TORI *taps on door number six. And they all nervously wait to be invited into* DOCTOR JULIAN'*s surgery.*

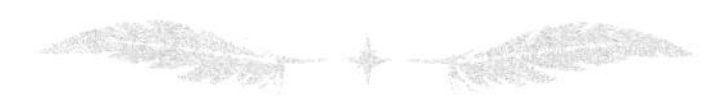

SCENE TWO

JULIAN (*breezily, whilst opening his surgery door*) Come in! (*He is immaculately dressed in a pale-blue shirt; navy tie; and navy trousers.*) (*Then to* JONATHAN, *politely*) You sit where you like. (JONATHAN *and* VICKI *enter the room with* TORI *close behind them. The bright, slightly cluttered surgery is well lit by two small sash windows and a low-level ceiling that is filled with the same halogen lamps seen in reception. Similarly, the cream coloured walls; brown-padded chairs; and light, beech-wood furnishings are equally familiar. There are a large number of wall sockets scattered around the room. A computer monitor rests on a small table. And a wide, oblong x-ray lamp fills the entire left-side wall.* JONATHAN *sits on a chair situated at the side of* JULIAN's *desk that is positioned beneath the window, far right.* VICKI *sits to* JONATHAN's *left. Whilst* TORI *sits on a chair that has been placed in the centre of the room so that she is directly facing both* JONATHAN *and* VICKI. *Because all four characters are aware that they are being filmed for the BBC's 'Cancer' documentary, they each fail to acknowledge* CAROLINE *and* MAX *who are discreetly positioned by the nearest window, door right. Along with* JACK, *who is now conspicuously poised behind his tripod and camera, far left.*) Right! When did I last see you?

VICKI You last saw us in January. We're late seeing you 'cos we went away, which we didn't suppose would make much difference.

JULIAN Nearly a month! (*Directly to* JONATHAN) What's the news?

JONATHAN Er, the news? Oh, I've got a few problems actually. One is my breathing (JONATHAN *sits bolt upright; takes a deep breath; and expands his chest*) – it's getting a bit difficult an' I don't wanna put it down to a chest infection 'cos it might not be that. And second is this lump in my shoulder (JONATHAN *lightly taps his left shoulder*) which

I would like you to have a little look at. It's getting like bigger.

JULIAN When did you notice that lump?

JONATHAN Er, I noticed … not a lump, I noticed it *hurting* about a couple of weeks ago: two an' a half, three weeks ago when it was just a pain in my shoulder. But now it's developed into a lump and it's …

JULIAN I don't think you mentioned *pain* last time I saw you.

JONATHAN No.

JULIAN So it's happened all in those few weeks?

JONATHAN Yeah.

JULIAN (*enquiringly*) And is it painful all the time?

JONATHAN Well, I know it's there 'cos I can *feel* it's there.

VICKI (*to* JONATHAN) And you said when you open and close doors and pick fings up.

JONATHAN Yeah. (JONATHAN *picks-up his bottle of natural spring water from* JULIAN*'s desk.*) That's alright. (*He puts the bottle back onto the desk and then picks up a small box of tissues.*) But fings like that an' moving them backwards (JONATHAN *rotates the box of tissues to his left.*)

JULIAN Yeah, okay. And you've not had anything like that before?

JONATHAN No.

JULIAN And you haven't injured yourself?

JONATHAN (*slowly, and very perceptively*) Yeah, I know… I've got an inclination of what it is but like you said …

JULIAN (*quickly*) You've got what?

JONATHAN An inclination to what it is but I s'pose …

JULIAN What do you *think* it is? (*Pause*) You presume it's related to the cancer?

JONATHAN Mmm … yeah.

JULIAN And you say you can feel something there?

JONATHAN It's a lump.

JULIAN (*casually*) Okay. I'll examine you in the examination room. (*Pause*) Tell me about your breathing.

JONATHAN Well, it's alright at the moment but when I go (JONATHAN *expands his chest again*) an' stick my chest out sometimes it's like a tightness around there (*he rubs the centre of his chest.*)

JULIAN (*inquisitively, to* JONATHAN) You're very conscious of your breathing?

JONATHAN Mmm.

JULIAN Okay. (*Pause*) Anything else?

JONATHAN They're the two main problems.

JULIAN You're otherwise feeling alright? (*Pause*) Eating?

JONATHAN Yeah.

JULIAN (*cautiously*) And, erm, how you feeling … generally?

JONATHAN (*quickly*) What d'yer mean? In my head?

(*Pause*)

JULIAN (*slowly*) Yeah. How's your head?

JONATHAN (*frankly*) I'm alright. I'm getting fings together. (*Pause*) I'm not lying to myself.

JULIAN *Not* lying to yourself?

JONATHAN Not lying to myself. No. Just trying to come to terms with the reality.

(*Pause*)

JULIAN *Is* there a temptation to lie to yourself?

JONATHAN (*softly*) No. Not really.

(*Pause*)

JULIAN (*slowly and deliberately*) And thoughts about … (*Pause, then quickly*) I mean, we talked a lot about treatment last time, Jonathan. Have you gone over any of that? Are there doubts about the decisions you've made?

JONATHAN Doubts? Na. I'm still going along with what I've said 'cos I fink it's best for me.

JULIAN Okay. (*He rises from his seat*) I'm gonna take you next door and exam you.

JONATHAN (*quietly, whilst rising from his seat*) Yeah; good.

(*There is a long pause whilst* JONATHAN *and* JULIAN *exit the room. And* VICKI *observes the big beech-wood door as it slowly closes behind them. She speaks to camera*):

RICHARD TOLD ME THAT JONATHAN is secretly planning a short break away with his friends. Good God! I hope he is kidding because it will be extremely difficult to tell him that he cannot possibly go. In truth, the harsh reality is that Jonathan now requires around the clock medical care and attention. Apart from severe breathing difficulties, he also suffers from excruciating leg cramps that often occur without warning and can last for several hours. Of course, Jonathan does not easily accept these facts because he only wants to live normally alongside his fun-loving friends for as long as he can. But, astonishingly, they still have no idea that he is terminally ill or even that he has had his foot amputated simply because Jonathan – against my own advice - has chosen not to tell them. I find it incredible! For sure, I will never forget those long-suffering hours I spent watching my wilful son as he practiced walking flawlessly in his new prosthesis. How he huffed and puffed; moaned and groaned; tripped and slipped until he eventually mastered it! I will also never forget the distressing morning when he hobbled off to school with just the aid of his dependable crutches and a temporary foot that was lightly held in place by a tiny piece of Velcro. I was horrified by his reckless behaviour. And, of course, I constantly pleaded with him not to be so foolish. However, as always, my stubborn son gave me no choice in the matter. So I had to bite my lip as I nervously watched him struggle up the road with a familiar look of fierce determination on his pale, young face that was equally admirable and disturbing. I sat by the telephone all morning. And, sure enough, sometime around midday I wept at the sound of Jonathan's panic-stricken voice as he pleaded with me to collect him from the telephone booth outside his school because his temporary foot had fallen off due to excessive use -

TORI (*patiently smiling at* VICKI) He speaks so well!

VICKI (*proudly*) All of my children do.

TORI Yeah. It's really impressive!

VICKI (*grinning widely*) Mmm … That's 'cos I used to speak to them a lot!

TORI (*laughing*) I can imagine that!

(*The two women briefly laugh together before* VICKI*'s light-hearted manner abruptly vanishes.*)

VICKI *I* need to speak with Julian about the treatment.

TORI Okay …

VICKI 'Cos, erm, the chemotherapy … (*then more quickly*) I know it's not gonna cure Jonathan but if it keeps it at bay …

TORI (*calmly*) It wouldn't necessarily do that. When Julian first worked out that he'd relapsed – when you came that time and it was unexpected – I think what Julian was trying to say, which is *exactly* what Jonathan picked-up, was that he couldn't guarantee whether it would have any effect. You know he said straight away: "It won't cure you."

VICKI We know that. But will it actually keep it … down.

TORI No. There's no guarantee of that.

VICKI That would be selfish of me to … But if I could get another six months with Jonathan. That's where we differ. He says, "No. I'm not gonna do that!" And I feel tempted to ask him.

TORI But how would you feel if he says, "Yes. It could possibly give you six months," and Jonathan's saying he doesn't want that?

VICKI How would I feel? (*Pause*) Well, there's no if's or but's about it: Jonathan won't do it an' that's it! He's his own man. He makes his own decisions an' I can't sway him.

TORI But that makes you …

(*Together*)

VICKI I could *try* …

TORI I *know* you could. That's why I'm asking you.

VICKI (*more to herself*) But that would be wrong.

(*Pause*)

TORI Yeah. But you *need* to know.

VICKI I need to know. Yeah. We did ask Julian before but it was … I don't want anyfing else but direct answers from him 'cos I can't really remember clearly if he said "it might", "maybe", or "not sure".

TORI I think I can remember what he said was "it *might*".

VICKI It might.

TORI But that's as far as he could go.

VICKI To Jonathan "might" is a "no". So …

TORI (*quickly*) Exactly! But you need to ask it. And Jonathan won't mind you asking again, will he? (*Lightly*) He'll probably *glare* at you for bringing it up!

VICKI Yeah. I know. We've spoken about it before we've come in an' I said, yer know, if he said "it might" would you do it and he's emphatic: it's a definite "No!"

TORI (*nodding*) Well, he's lucky Vicki 'cos he's got a mum who will respect what *he* wants. Where it gets difficult sometimes is if you've got a mum that wants the opposite to what their child wants and that puts the child under pressure to perhaps do something that they don't want to do. But they do it for their mother; whereas you wouldn't put him under that pressure. But it *does* put you in a very difficult position 'cos you're left with – when you *do* loose Jonathan – "I *could* have had him for longer!" And that's hard for you 'cos an extra *hour* is important for you.

(*Pause*)

VICKI Having last year an' seeing other parents, and patients, dealing with the same situation we're in an', erm, they're like screaming an' pulling their hair out … It's all to no avail! I've seen it. I *know* how it works.

TORI You mean searching for different treatments?

VICKI Searching for anything. Any hope. *Give* 'em anything. *Do* anyfing you can just to get that little bit longer with them. And probably the chemo's had no effect at all anyway. It's just made the child very, very sick in a situation when they really should be just enjoying ev'ry day for what it is.

TORI There's different reasons for giving chemotherapy. Sometimes the hope is to hold the disease at bay, like you say, or to give them a bit longer. Sometimes if someone is very symptomatic sometimes having chemotherapy *sometimes* can help allay some of the symptoms. But there's always a buy-off between the side-effects of the chemotherapy versus what it's going to do in certain situations. (*Pause*) So I think it's just important to ask Julian that question and have it answered honestly for you.

VICKI Yeah. (*Pause*) I kinda know what he's gonna say but I need to ask it.

TORI (*quickly*) Just like if there was something on the news tomorrow that was a miracle drug you'd still need to phone-up and check it wasn't suitable for Jonathan. Maybe if it was suddenly said that it works effectively with Synovial Sarcomas you'd need to check it out!

VICKI He knows he's really, really sick an' there's nothing … there's no hope an' nuffing they can do for him an' his way of thinking is: "Why make me even worse!"

TORI But what's interesting in what you said there, Vicki, is when you say, "There's no hope." (*Quickly*) Just knowing how Jonathan is and how *you* are … I know there's no hope of him being cured but what you and Jonathan have shown is that you've actually found some way of making the most of what you've got, haven't you? You haven't given-up. Although he might not be having treatment, which some people might see as giving-up. Do you see what I mean? But what Jonathan's doing is living his life, isn't he?

VICKI Well, yeah. Ev'ry single day is precious an' he doesn't want to spend it in our local hospital having blood transfusions. And he doesn't want his hair falling out. And vomiting. And not eating. And not being wiv his friends. He wants to …

TORI He wants to be Jonathan!

VICKI He does! He doesn't want to give-up until he *has* to give-up an' that's what the chemo would make him do.

TORI Yeah. But some people would think that *not* having treatment is giving-up whereas I'd say it's the opposite. What he's doing is *living* despite the awful things that he's got to face.

VICKI Well, I'm glad you've said that 'cos there's quite a lot of people who are actually making me feel quite guilty. I've had phone calls from people saying, yer know, "There's *this* doctor: Try this – we'll pay for you". And "Are you doing enough? You seem *so* calm about all this!" They make me feel guilty. And yet they know *nuffing* about Jonathan's cancer or anyfing about what we've gone through privately an' how we've come to this partnership between us where we've decided … .

TORI (*softly*) Mmm … you're *respecting* him, aren't you?

VICKI Yeah. Not going out screaming my head off. Just valuing him and the time I've got wiv him.

TORI (*quickly*) And often people that are phoning you saying, "Have you tried this, that and the other" is because *they* can't deal with what you and Jonathan have been forced to face. But at the end of the day you'll never go against him in any way because you respect him so much.

VICKI Well, I trust Julian too. I trust that Julian would definitely do ev'ryfing he could for him.

TORI (*softly*) He would. But the people that are phoning you are the ones that *don't* know the situation and haven't been through what you've been through. People *might* even know. They might have seen Jonathan without his hair but they don't know what's happened at home: what you've gone through privately.

VICKI (*incidentally*) Well, they haven't seen him wivout his hair! (*The two women laugh aloud*) No-one's seen him wivout his hair! He had a hat on day an' night!

TORI People *think* they know but they don't.

VICKI And they say, "We don't know what to say, really." An' I go, "Well, don't *say* anyfing! If you can't say anything supportive please just don't say anyfing!" 'Cos it just makes me feel bad when they start saying, yer know (*she mimics speech*): "Don't give-up hope. Try this.

Try that." Hang on! This is *my* child and maybe the last few months he's got left to live! I'm not gonna put him through all that just to be seen to be doing summink!

(*Pause*)

TORI It takes a huge amount of courage both on Jonathan's behalf - and yours - to be able to stick with what Jonathan's decided when you've got all these people saying all these sorts of things.

(*Pause*)

VICKI (*suddenly and very sombrely*) I need to talk to you about, erm, the immediate future … what's gonna happen 'cos I really only wanna live for today. But I'm forced to kinda ask you a few questions.

TORI I think when Julian comes back in with Jonathan we need to have a look at that x-ray and that will give us some information. Jonathan's having more breathing difficulties that I think it's probably, realistically, that his chest disease has got bigger.

VICKI (*softly*) I'm *dreading* that.

TORI (*sympathetically*) I know.

VICKI I'm dreading it!

TORI Do you think about it a lot?

VICKI All the time! You open yer eyes an' you fink about it. You go to bed *finking* about it. *When* will the symptoms start? When will, yer know, will it all happen?

TORI And we don't often see death so close-up, do we?

VICKI It's hard for me to imagine.

(*Pause*)

TORI And what you were saying is the reason why you can't look too far ahead is that you've got a responsibility for *now*, which is looking after him *now*. And each day your responsibility will change slightly with what happens. But you can't think too far ahead otherwise you wouldn't be able to function as well as you're functioning now, which I'm sure is taking a huge amount of effort at times.

VICKI Yeah. But you do it. *I* can be strong if *he's* strong and *he's* strong if I'm strong. (*Pause*) 'Cos I was crying all over the place, as yer know, an' he said he understood that 'cos if the boot was on the other foot he would be the same. But when he asked me, yer know, "Mum. Can you stop crying for *me* an' just be strong for *me*?" Then you've just gotta do that!

(*Long pause*)

TORI He's very much his own person, isn't he?

VICKI Of course!

(*The conversation between the two women abruptly ends when* JONATHAN *and* JULIAN *re-enter the room. And as they return to their vacant seats,* VICKI *observes the big beech-wood door as it slowly closes behind them. She speaks to camera*):

THERE IS NOTHING I TREASURE more than spending a nice quiet day alone with Jonathan. Indeed, we still laugh and joke around as much as ever. And even when we're busy doing separate things, I still gain a tremendous sense of inner-peace and contentment simply from experiencing the warm, powerful bond that has always existed between us.

"Let's pretend to be out when Flora calls!" Jonathan

humorously said, as we ate our lunch together last Friday. I smiled at his childish request. "No. Seriously mum." He continued. "Just for today, I'd really like to forget that I've got cancer."

Nonetheless, when I opened our front door to his Home-Care nurse just a short while later, my placid son became uncharacteristically short-tempered with us both. I was shocked by his severe mood swing. But, in truth, it was my own angry response towards him that disturbed me the most. Indeed, once Flora had gone Jonathan and I continued to bicker for a short while longer before he eventually sulked off to play on his computer. Meanwhile, I cried alone inside our run-down kitchen feeling deeply sad and remorseful for having upset my brave and fearless son who has, to date, done nothing but his utmost to protect me from his own intense suffering. For several minutes, my head hung in shame. Then, to my complete surprise, I felt Jonathan's silent presence standing close behind me. He caused me to almost jump out of my skin because it was as though he had emerged from nowhere. Of course, my mischievous son was grinning from ear to ear at having startled me so badly. And I soon laughed too. Then, without another word, we hugged each other for a long time. However, when he eventually returned to his computer game I, once again, sobbed alone simply because only God knows how much I will miss my cherished son after he is gone. In truth, the only thing that is holding me together during this difficult time is my steadfast faith in the strength of the human spirit, along with my certain knowledge that Jonathan and I can never be wholly parted.

SCENE THREE

JULIAN (*factually, to* VICKI) O.K. Sorry. Jonathan *has* got a lump there, as he says. While I can't be a hundred per cent certain that it's cancer it seems quite *likely*, even though that's a relatively *unusual* way for this cancer to behave. But, actually, you get a lump that's painful; it's grown over that sort of time; that's the most likely thing.

VICKI A cyst moves, doesn't it? A tumour doesn't. An' *that* doesn't move.

JONATHAN Yeah. But isn't it a coincidence that I get a cyst right now?

JULIAN Yeah. Exactly. (*Hesitantly*) I don't think that we can be a hundred per cent certain but I certainly think we can decide what we *do* about it on the basis that it *is* cancer. The way I would approach something like this is to think about whether it should be removed. Okay? And the reason for removing it is because that's quite a quick, simple and straightforward thing to do in which we can take it out; put it in a bucket; you heal up quite quickly; and the problem's done. Okay?

VICKI What about his lungs, though? Having an operation like that …

JULIAN (*to* JONATHAN) I don't think there's a problem for you from the point-of-view of your lungs because again – and I've said it before – most of your lungs are still fine. Okay? The disease in your lungs *has* changed from a month ago …

VICKI (*quickly*) Have you looked?

JULIAN Yep.

VICKI (*quickly*) Drastically?

JULIAN No. It's changed but not drastically. First, I'm not sure how much of the breathlessness you're noticing, and so on, is *really* related to the change in your lung disease. I mean, you're gonna be very conscious of your breathing, I'm sure, aren't you? But it hasn't, sort of, dramatically changed. And second, your lungs are nowhere near the situation where we think, "Oh, it would be dangerous to have an operation."

JONATHAN The fing is, I've put all that – the operations an' being in hospital wiv the needles in me an' ev'ryfing – I've put all that behind me and I just wanted to say, like: "That's the last of my operations and my last time of being laid-up in a hospital bed!"

JULIAN I understand. And if you've done that it's difficult because there isn't a way you can do an operation without it *being* like an operation. And if there's a bit of you that just feels, you know, that you just can't stand the idea of going in there; lying in a gown; going to theatre; and all that sort of thing …

JONATHAN But it's not *just* that. It's just the feeling of … I get the worry an' the … just ev'ryfing about it I put behind me.

JULIAN What: going to sleep and … ?

JONATHAN Yeah. I don't want to re-live it. All that anaesthetic going into me …

JULIAN (*sympathetically*) Because it's like … like your amputation? (JONATHAN *visibly cringes as* JULIAN *says the word 'amputation'. This is followed by a very long, uneasy silence.*) *Is* it because of that?

JONATHAN (*irritated, to* CAROLINE) I should have had a word wiv him, shouldn't I?

CARO (*encouragingly*) It's alright. We can cut that out. You just go on, Jonny.

JONATHAN (*politely, to* JULIAN) Just don't mention that again.

JULIAN (*slightly embarrassed*) Alright. But … like *that* operation, I mean, the operations that you remember before.

JONATHAN How big do you fink it is by feeling it?

JULIAN A couple of centimetres.

JONATHAN (*surprised*) Really? Is *that* it? (JULIAN *nods*) It feels a lot bigger than that to me!

VICKI (*to* JULIAN) He doesn't have to make a decision now, does he?

JONATHAN (*quickly, to* VICKI) I'm not gonna decide now.

VICKI (*suddenly and very directly, to* JULIAN) Julian. I've gotta ask this again. I've asked it before an' it's still not clear in my head an' I kinda know what your answers gonna be but I have to just ask – a direct answer: If he has more chemo, the Iphosomide, is it – in your professional opinion – likely to keep this cancer at bay and prolong Jonathan's illness, or is it just … not gonna do nuffing?

JONATHAN (*exasperated, to* VICKI) Haven't we gone through this already?

VICKI (*apologetically*) I *know* but it kind of …

TORI (*quickly, to* JONATHAN) Yeah. But she needs to ask.

VICKI (*to* JULIAN) I just need to know, yer know … honestly.

JULIAN If you're concerned about there being *a big* missed opportunity for Jonathan …

VICKI Not a big missed opportunity. But if I could keep him longer

… .

JULIAN (*holding his chin*) I have to say I don't think it would make a major difference. And actually, you know, I'm influenced by … by this lump appearing …

VICKI (*quickly*) What d'yer mean *influenced*?

JULIAN Well, just because I think that's a mark of the way his disease is behaving, which is slightly different from what we knew up until now. Erm, it's not just a disease that's confined to his lungs. I think that's a graver situation if you like.

VICKI See! I remember saying to you that he must have a tumour somewhere else for his lungs to get like this once the main site had been removed. There were no signs of this. But, obviously, that's what's happened … *I* feel.

JULIAN I don't think the things have come into his lungs from there.

VICKI You don't?

JULIAN No. I think it's part and parcel of the same process.

VICKI Do you?

JULIAN Yeah.

VICKI (*resignedly*) Okay. (*Pause, then incidentally*) So, that's not a direct … that's a 'No'.

JULIAN That's a 'No'.

TORI (*to* VICKI) That's very direct, isn't it?

VICKI Well you need to be, don't yer?

JONATHAN (*sarcastically*) Never seen you act like that before!

(TORI *half laughs*)

JULIAN I'll just do it again: No!

VICKI That's fine. I *knew* that but last time it was like "maybe" "if" and "perhaps". But a definite "no" is a bit different from them words, innit?

JULIAN (*looking out of the window and visibly struggling under* VICKI*'s directness*) You know, is that a sunny day or a cloudy day? It's quite hard! And yet, what *I* don't want to do is to suddenly, you know, close-off options. I have to think each time I see you what can I be doing for the best for you. And that depends on the circumstances. But in terms of how much is Jonathan missing out in terms of having intensive chemotherapy in the light of all the treatment that he's had up until now? The answer is that I just *don't* think it would make a substantial difference.

VICKI He would be missing out on a lot of living if he had that chemo so …

JULIAN (*quietly*) He certainly would.

VICKI (*to* JONATHAN) He knows that, don't yer?

JONATHAN Exactly. That's right. That's partly what made me make my decisions.

VICKI (*to* JULIAN) He doesn't wanna be in here or our local hospital and stuck in bed an' sick for no reason. (*Pause*) That's it!

JONATHAN (*to* JULIAN) Did you look at the x-rays yet?

JULIAN (*to* JONATHAN) I've looked at the x-rays.

JONATHAN And what d'yer reckon on that then?

JULIAN I think the x-rays show that your disease *has* got a bit worse over the past month. I've tried to sort of link that with the symptoms that you've noticed in terms of your breathlessness and I would still say that I, you know, I don't think your symptoms of breathlessness are because your disease has suddenly got a lot worse. I think a part of that is because you're going to be very conscious of your breathing at the moment.

JONATHAN (*adamantly*) I don't think it is! I mean, I could tell the difference if it was like just in my head: if I was just conscious of it. Even if I didn't know there was anyfing wrong with me I'd still think there was summink wrong 'cos I can just *feel* it.

JULIAN I'm not saying that you wouldn't notice anything but what I'm trying to say is that, you know, your lungs *have* deteriorated a bit over that time but it's not dramatic.

JONATHAN You think it's partly psychosomatic then?

JULIAN (*defensively*) I'm not saying it's psychosomatic at all. I'm saying that if you're worried that your breathing is more difficult and, therefore, everything that your chest x-ray … I mean, I can show you your chest x-ray if it helps.

JONATHAN Yeah. Would you?

VICKI (*to* JONATHAN) You sure you wanna look at these?

JONATHAN (*softly*) Yeah. It's alright.

(JULIAN *rises from his chair. He crosses the room whilst taking* JONATHAN*'s recent x-rays out of a large, brown envelope. He pins them onto the wide, oblong lamp situated on the left-side wall before switching it on.* TORI *promptly moves into* JULIAN*'s vacant chair to avoid blocking* JONATHAN*'s view.*)

JULIAN (*pointing to one of the x-rays*) O.K. That's today's chest x-ray.

VICKI (*to* JONATHAN) D'yer wanna get closer?

JONATHAN Yeah. I wanna ask him summink. (*Pause*) What's that thing down there, Julian? (JONATHAN *points*) That bit there.

JULIAN That's, erm, just gas in your bowel.

(JONATHAN *grins at* VICKI *and she laughs aloud.*) (*She speaks to camera*):

SOMETIMES IT'S HARD TO ACCEPT that Jonathan is no longer fighting for his life but only for a dignified death. But, in truth, we both know our arduous battle against cancer ended a long time ago. And yet it is also true that we still possess a strange sense of hope for the immediate future. Of course, it is not the kind of hope we once knew. We no longer hope for a new treatment that will instantly cure Jonathan. And we longer hope for some divine intervention to miraculously bring about his full recovery. No. Those days of believing that Jonathan would be one of the lucky ones who would sail through his treatment and survive against all the odds simply because he was young, vibrant and exceptionally strong are well and truly behind us. Without doubt, he's always been a fighter and so have I. And at the start of his illness Jonathan certainly put up an admirable fight for his life knowing that - at fourteen - he had so much to live for. Yet, in hindsight, I cannot deny that the truth about his illness was always out there. Even during those early days when Jonathan first arrived on the Cancer Unit.

"I'd like to go in by myself," he told me, as we sat inside the waiting area of the Cardiology Department where his heart was to be tested to determine he was strong enough to withstand chemotherapy treatment. I was surprised at Jonathan's sudden request but happily agreed he could go it alone. As I waited for him to re-join me, I grew increasingly restless. I read the medical posters on the clinic wall several times over; I fidgeted in my seat when the other patients caught me observing them much too closely; finally, I casually flicked through Jonathan's medical notes that we carried with us from clinic to clinic. Unsurprisingly, Doctor Julian's handwriting was extremely difficult to decipher. But when I concentrated *really* hard on the tiny black letters that were messily scrawled across the top of the first page, I almost fell off my seat when I slowly read *Met ... as ... tas ... es.* Instantly, an alarm bell rang inside my head. Followed by my own shell-shocked voice inwardly screeching *NO WAY!* I wanted to shout *HOW CAN THIS BE!!*? to the kind nurse sitting at reception. And yet, presented with the absolute truth about Jonathan's illness all I could do was stare into space like a stuffed dummy. Whilst my scrambled mind desperately tried to make sense out of the startling information it had just received. I must have looked a dreadful state when Jonathan re-joined me:

"What's up, mum?" He constantly asked, as we made our way back to the ward.

"Absolutely nuffing, babes: I'm just *really* tired today." I repeatedly told him, in a light and breezy manner.

But I knew that Jonathan knew that I was lying. Oh, God! How I struggled with my dark and sinister thoughts later that same evening. It felt like a living hell. And yet, curiously, I awoke the following morning feeling surprisingly positive about Jonathan's immediate future. Indeed, somehow my over-wrought mind had succeeded in erasing all of my deepest fears from the night before. *I will NOT believe anything negative unless Julian tells me otherwise* became my new-found affirmation. It really was as simple as that! -

VICKI (*to* JONATHAN) Is there anyfing else you need to ask?

JULIAN (*to* JONATHAN, *with a slight hint of impatience*) What else?

JONATHAN Have you got anything else to say?

JULIAN No.

JONATHAN (*to* VICKI) What about you?

(*There is a long pause.* JONATHAN *and* VICKI *stare at each other. She is clearly thinking about her next question.*)

VICKI (*suddenly, to* JULIAN) You know the bigger it gets – the tumour? The main tumour.

JULIAN (*clutching his chin more tightly*) Yeah …

VICKI The bigger it gets and the longer it goes on … the *quicker* it grows, dunnit? Because each cell divides ev'ry three weeks so the more cells you've got the quicker that's gonna get bigger. D'yer know what I'm saying? It might take …

JULIAN Well … it's gonna *look* bigger and bigger …

VICKI But it's gonna be even more … rapid. As the weeks go on. As it gets bigger.

JONATHAN Yeah. *I* know what yer mean.

VICKI The main tumour. (*To* JONATHAN) *You* know what I'm saying? (*To* JULIAN) *That's* what I wanna know. It's true, innit?

JULIAN Well, tumours tend to grow at a steady rate but their rate of growth *can* change …

VICKI His is high-grade though, innit?

JULIAN (*hesitantly*) Yeah … What's behind your question? What's your concern?

JONATHAN (*to* VICKI) *I* know what you're getting at.

VICKI (*to* JONATHAN) Yeah. What … (*Pause*)

(*Together*)

JONATHAN No. Leave it.

VICKI (*more to herself*) No. Leave it. (*To* JULIAN, *dismissively*) No. It's okay. (*Pause*) No. We'll see you again anyway, won't we?

JULIAN (*smiling*) I hope so! I'm happy to see you.

VICKI (*suddenly, to* JONATHAN) D'yer want me to leave the room?

JONATHAN (*surprised*) Why?

VICKI Is there anyfing you want to speak to Julian privately about?

JONATHAN No. I don't think there is. Nuffing I can't ask him without you being there anyway.

JULIAN (*kindly*) Jonathan. I'm happy to talk to you and if, you know, if you want to speak it doesn't have to be now. Okay?

JONATHAN Yeah.

VICKI (*picking-up* JONATHAN*'s jacket in preparation to leave*) Yeah. Thank you, Julian.

TORI (*to* VICKI) Er, *we* can talk can't we? I think Julian …

JULIAN (*rising from his chair*) I'll see you in a couple of weeks' time.

VICKI You don't need your room for anyfing?

JULIAN No. I'm done with it. (*He scoops-up a large pile of medical notes from his desk and puts them under his left arm.*) Right. I'm off.

Bye all!

VICKI Thank you very much.

JONATHAN Thank you.

TORI (*to* JONATHAN) Now. Do we want to talk together, or separate?

(JULIAN *exits the room. And* VICKI *observes the big beech-wood door as it slowly closes behind him. She speaks to camera*):

LOOKING BACK, I AM TRULY amazed by how strong and resourceful we have all been so far. Indeed, I almost laugh when I recall the intense distress I felt at seeing Jonathan being wheeled off to theatre simply to have his Hickman Line fitted. His chemotherapy treatment hadn't even begun! But I honestly think neither of us could have coped with too much information during those early stages in his illness. Even so, I am still surprised by how we found the necessary strength to cope with each new phase as it unfolded. Like the time we first experienced the shocking side-effects of his chemotherapy treatment. Typically, Jonathan's body temperature soared during the middle of the night. He could barely move a limb. And yet, to my dismay, it took me several hours to convince him that his life was in danger and that he needed to visit our local hospital straight away.

"Let me find you a wheelchair," I insisted, when I saw he had no strength to walk through the cold, winding corridors of the Greenwich District Hospital.

"I'm *not* getting into one of those fings!" Jonathan defiantly hissed back at me.

And so, as usual, I had to bite my lip as my wilful son desperately attempted to soldier-on to the paediatric ward completely unaided. And in that exact moment, I thought my heart would burst into a thousand little pieces from the overwhelming sympathy I felt for Jonathan. Then, when he finally collapsed like a two year old toddler onto the hospital's hard and dusty floor, I quickly panicked. It was around 3 a.m. There was not a soul in sight. My panic soon increased when I had no choice but to abandon him in the hope of finding an available nurse or suitable wheelchair. Indeed, Jonathan was so angry and humiliated by his unexpected defeat. And yet we could never have known this was just the first of many more equally humiliating moments to come. Like the time when he was advised to have his sperm frozen in case his treatment caused him to become infertile. Eventually, we both managed to laugh about this particularly embarrassing subject but, at fourteen, it was not easy for Jonathan to cope with. Then there was the time when Richard and Daniel asked me to shave their own heads when their brother's lovely locks began to fall out by the handful. I thought it admirable of them and I know Jonathan greatly appreciated their support. But he could not hide his deep-rooted sadness knowing, unlike Richard and Daniel, his own much loved hair would not return within the foreseeable future. And then there was the time when a doctor at our local hospital almost fainted on the spot when Jonathan began to vomit huge clumps of bright-red blood due to some internal bleeding that went undetected over several days. However, humiliation aside, without doubt the most significant moment in Jonathan's illness, to date, will always be when Julian told us he had relapsed in his lungs. Because until that ominous day last January, we all believed my proud and fearless son was still fighting for his life. Then, in an instant, he wasn't. Naturally, he was severely scarred by his chemotherapy treatment. And his amputation is another story. But prior to that inauspicious morning, we had every reason to believe that the worst of Jonathan's illness was all behind us. Then the lightning struck. And unimaginable fear coupled with extreme sadness suddenly replaced our naïve optimism. In the blink of an eye, our blind and constant hope that my much loved second son would have a bright and happy future with his loving family was cruelly snatched away from us. In truth, there are no words to describe the intense grief I felt when I witnessed Jonathan hit that brick wall sending him straight back to square one. From there on, all I could do for him was pray.

Scene closes to 'When You Believe'
sung by Whitney Houston and Mariah Carey.

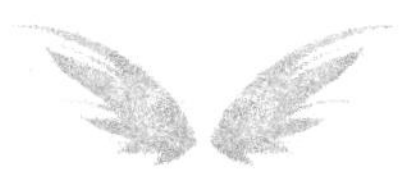

ACT THREE

Make Me Smile

Introducing

DOCTOR GUY, a renowned Palliative Care Consultant. Medium height; stocky build; warm-grey eyes; and balding grey hair. Casual, confident and caring. He wears a heavy silver watch on his right wrist and a tight-fitting copper bracelet on his left. A picture identity card on a silver chain hangs loosely around his neck. He constantly peeps over the top of his silver-rimmed glasses that are resting on the tip of his plump nose and is discreetly chewing on a small piece of gum throughout. He has a forthright, down-to-earth manner and a standard London accent.

FLORA, a Homecare Community Nurse employed by the London Borough of Greenwich. Small and curvaceous; dark-brown eyes; and short, dark-brown hair. Highly practical, efficient and supportive. Her over-sized, rimless glasses cover most of her tiny features. She wears no jewellery except for a black watch on her left wrist. And although normally very chatty, due to the presence of the BBC crew she is unusually quiet and self-conscious. Consequently, her deliberate speech is humorously slow and exaggerated. She is overtly timid and has a soft London accent.

Setting: A cosy side-room situated close to the Cancer Unit in a busy central London hospital.

SCENE ONE

10th May, 2001: *It is mid-afternoon. Due to a rapid decline in his health, JONATHAN (wearing a long-sleeve blue and white check shirt; beige trousers; and navy trainers) and VICKI (wearing a long-sleeve cerise tee-shirt; black trousers; and white trainers) have arrived at the Cancer Unit to discuss his forthcoming palliative care. In a cosy side-room close to the Unit, they are both seated on a small, navy sofa that rests against the near-side wall, door left. The overcrowded room is newly decorated with cream coloured walls; dark-green paint; and light-blue carpet. On the farthest wall, opposite the door, a radiator sits beneath two sash windows. They are firmly closed. And yet, they fail to block-out the rumbling road-works coming from the street below. CAROLINE, JACK, and MAX are busy organising the set before filming. Whilst GUY (wearing a white, short-sleeve shirt; red tie; blue trousers; and black shoes), TORI (wearing a navy blouse; beige skirt; and black shoes), and FLORA (wearing a blue roll-neck jumper; cropped black trousers; and black pumps) are all strategically seated in a neat semi-circle around the small sofa. But their loud, superfluous conversations wash over VICKI who stretches-out her arms and yawns as though she were alone. Suddenly smiling, she speaks to camera*:

RICHARD AND JONATHAN HAVE ALWAYS shared the same sense of humour, which can be very funny sometimes. Indeed, only today - whilst standing on the platform of our local train station - Jonathan became highly amused when he spotted Richard sitting on our shabby-pink sofa whilst watching television from inside our tiny front-room. He quickly rang his super-relaxed brother from his mobile phone:

"Rick! Go to the kitchen window!" He ordered, playfully.

Of course, Richard - who was visibly surprised at being spotted from such a distance - did as Jonathan asked. Then the two boys frantically waved to each other in a silly and childish fashion before Jonathan humorously continued:

"Now jump up and down like a monkey! And pull stupid faces at the same time!

And to Jonathan's extreme delight Richard, once again, did not hesitate to do as he was asked. My goodness, it was truly wonderful to hear Jonathan laugh so heartily. To top it all, ridiculous Richard continued to jump, wave and pull stupid monkey faces right up until our train arrived approximately ten minutes later -

GUY (*impatiently, to* JACK) Are you guys recording now? (*He turns to* FLORA.) So Jonathan at home: What's your normal pattern of practice?

FLORA (*nervously*) Armm, we use the tertiary hospital and the local, armm, but I think with Jonathan, you know, you've got this, armm, link with the, armm, with the Greenwich and Bexley Hospice as well. So I'm hoping that they can, armm …

GUY 'Cos that's what I wanted to be clear about. (*Pause. He turns to* VICKI) I think the essential thing is to put together a package that works for *you*. I mean, in a sense you almost haven't got to have any evidence of us being around so that you guys can do *what* you want *when* you want. And from a practical point of view, being at home - one of the things that *is* important, I think, is being able to get hold of people out of hours 'cos if things are going to hit the fan they do it …

JONATHAN They always happen at night.

GUY Exactly! They do it when you least need it and when you're least prepared.

VICKI (*coolly*) We've experienced that already. (*She speaks to camera*):

ANYHOW, EVERYONE WAS UP EARLY today except for me. In fact, to my surprise, Jonathan woke me with a nice morning cuppa. Then he sat on the end of my bed and happily chatted like he always did before he became ill with cancer. Now all I can think about is those hectic school-run days when Jonathan's biggest concern in life was no more than whether he had enough deodorant or peppermint gum to last him throughout the day! However, he further surprised me when - just prior to leaving the house – he bluntly commented on my physical appearance:

"Your face looks different," he said, as I applied some make-up.

"What d'yer mean *different*?" I hurriedly asked.

Jonathan paused for a brief moment before he continued:

"Oh, I dunno … *harder* I s'pose, especially wiv the lipstick. It don't suit yer. You look much better … *natural*."

"Well, cheers big ears! You've done my confidence the world of good!" I joked.

And we both laughed. But, inwardly, I understood exactly what Jonathan was trying to say. Because now, whenever I catch sight of myself in a mirror or shop window, I often cringe at my altered features. It's true, my eyes *do* seem smaller; my cheekbones sharper; and my mouth more taut and thinner too. And yet, what astounds me the most is the undeniable fact that no matter how hard we may try to keep up appearances, it is nigh on impossible to hide our true selves from those who know us really well -

GUY (*to* VICKI) And so, the essential thing, really, is making sure that you've got access to support.

FLORA (*quickly, but quietly*) We also use Marie Curie nurses as well – to suit. Obviously, they can't do any drug changes or administer drugs but they sit with the families, armm …

TORI (*to* JONATHAN) Do you understand what that means, Jonathan? The 'Marie Curie' nurses? It could be someone who could be there *if* you felt you wanted it. Not everybody does.

JONATHAN I know what they are.

GUY (*nodding, to* FLORA) Right. And do you normally work with the Bexley team if people are dying at home?

FLORA Armm, with the younger children, armm, it tends to be the tertiary hospital and the local consultants. Armm, but with the older children we alert the Greenwich and Bexley Hospice.

GUY (*still nodding to Flora*) Right. So one of the things that would be a good idea is for you to get a chance to talk to them and see what you want to do. As far as I'm concerned, we will plug any gaps that are necessary. (*He turns to* JONATHAN) And that's really a phone support that we can provide to you. If you actually need someone to come out from Palliative Care then it needs to be the local team. And actually, if you've got an established relationship with them then that's good, then either you or they can ring me if there's a problem or you're unsure about something because as I understand, Vicki, it's working quite well for you getting support from them?

VICKI The problem I've got is that Jonathan wants to be at home as much as possible. What's actually happening is all this help that's around is actually gonna be needed *within* the home – not *outside* the home. (*She turns to* JONATHAN) I'm right in that, yeah?

JONATHAN (*softly nodding*) Yeah. (VICKI *speaks to camera*):

THE INTENSE STRESS SURROUNDING JONATHAN'S illness has drastically altered the atmosphere inside our family home. Although I cannot recall exactly when the change took place, I do know that in Jonathan's pre-cancer days my four rowdy children would laugh, bicker and quarrel together. And now they don't. In fact, some days I hardly recognise where I live! But, in truth, I miss their raised voices; bedroom doors being slammed so hard the whole house would shudder; and even those occasional flying objects that would unexpectedly soar through the air whenever a sudden fit of temper spiralled out of control. Naturally, the children believe they are helping me by being so quiet. And they are. But their subdued silence secretly disturbs me far more than any teenage tantrum ever could. Yet, sadly, they each fail to recognise in their controlled efforts to remain 'normal' for Jonathan's sake they are not being normal at all! Moreover, realising that I am incapable of meeting the emotional needs of all my children at this difficult time has filled me with tremendous worry and guilt. Regardless, for now, Jonathan remains my top priority and his welfare must come before anything else -

GUY (*to* JONATHAN) Well, being at home is where you should be, you know, if that's where you wanna be.

JONATHAN That's where I wanna be.

VICKI (*slightly pleading*) But I'm worried 'cos he doesn't tell me fings until the last minute 'cos he just *doesn't* complain. And then we get this breathing difficulty where he can't breathe in the night an' I have to rush him to hospital. It was like three hours later that I realised how serious his symptoms were. I don't want the responsibility of having to judge what's the right thing to do with the medication – what to give; what *not* to give – 'cos he tries to do as much as he can for himself and *sometimes* he might get it wrong. Then it falls on my shoulders an' that's when I need outside support.

GUY (*to* JONATHAN) How do you feel about this: *you* being in control of the situation? Do you think it's your mum being anxious?

JONATHAN Erm, I can see what she means about not wanting the responsibility of judging. (*To* VICKI, *kindly*) I can see what you mean about it.

VICKI (*to* JONATHAN) 'Cos even your medications: you like to have them by yer bedside; you like to take them when *you* feel you need them. But sometimes you might need a different type of medication and then you won't let me interfere or give my opinion. (*To GUY*) An' sometimes he doesn't know when it might be the right time to change.

GUY (*to* JONATHAN) Is this a bloke thing, do you think?

JONATHAN I don't think so. I think it's an individual fing.

TORI (*to* JONATHAN, *quickly*) But Jonathan. We also respect you. I know him well enough, he'd say: "Well, if Jonathan wants to be in control he can be in control – to a certain point." But on the other hand that means that you *do* have to partake in some of these difficult conversations 'cos already today - I'm already *a bit* concerned that we should be able to make your pain better.

JONATHAN You are?

TORI (*quickly*) Yeah. But what I'm saying is that means us having that conversation which is what's difficult for you and which is why it's much easier to have it with mum. Do you see what I mean? But that puts pressure on mum and on both of you. So it's important. In one way it's better to have a conversation together.

JONATHAN (*compliantly*) Yeah. Yeah.

VICKI My point, Tori, really is 'cos Jonathan's been so brilliant in handling his illness as much as he can for himself, he does deserve the respect of dealing even with this stage as much as possible too.

TORI (*sympathetically*) Of course.

VICKI (*quickly*) And yet he *might* get it wrong an' I don't want him to get it wrong and be in any unnecessary pain at the same time. That's where I'm … (*She speaks to camera*):

I WAS REALLY WORRIED ABOUT Jonathan after he complained of severe breathing difficulties soon after he returned home from seeing his friends last Monday. He had just finished eating his evening meal when, after much fuss, he reluctantly admitted experiencing similar trouble throughout the day. However, because it is easy to confuse asthma with a chest infection, or possibly something worse, I decided to ask Jonathan outright about his private meeting with Julian which he attended last Friday. Cosily sitting together on our shabby- pink sofa, I tentatively began:

"Jon. You know that meeting wiv Julian, well … did you ask him about the tumours in yer lungs?"

Agitated by my direct manner, Jonathan's left knee bounced up and down. And as his large, hazel eyes glared back at me from inside his ghostly pale complexion, I saw his overwhelming desire to protect me from the truth. A solid lump rose inside my throat.

"Yeah, mum, I did." He finally admitted. "I looked at my new x-rays 'cos I needed to see how much bigger the tumours have grown. But I don't want you to worry."

A black silence filled the room. It soon crushed me. Broken, I openly wept into my cupped hands partly out of sympathy for Jonathan and partly out of sheer respect for the tremendous consideration he had shown towards me. I held his hands in mine:

"Jon. We both know this ain't gonna be easy." I cried. "But you'll *never* be on your own. I promise. An' ev'ryone will do their best to make fings easy for you especially me." I kissed his familiar hands. "You're just *so* special Jonny an' I'm gonna miss you more than you'll *ever* know! But one day we *will* be together again. I know it! And not just me, Jon, but *ev'ry* single person you know will be wiv you again 'cos no-one lives forever. Not no-one."

Jonathan's eyes filled with tears. I held him close. And, together, we fell into a new golden silence.

"Mum." he eventually whispered. "I'm *not* afraid to die. Honestly. I just wish it wasn't *so* painful."

"And I wish wiv all my heart that I could take it from you, darling. But I *can't*!" I cried again.

Jonathan and I spoke no more. Still cosily huddled together on our shabby-pink sofa, we returned into the golden silence. And we stayed there for a long time -

GUY (*sympathetically*) Have you got any actual fears, Jonathan? Are there any things that are worrying you about being at home and having your medication and running a lot of it yourself?

JONATHAN I s'pose the fing that worries me the most is becoming in a painful situation at home, say at three o'clock in the morning, an' not knowing what to do about it.

GUY So one of *our* jobs is to make sure that you know how to use your medications and what you've got available.

JONATHAN That's it. Yeah.

VICKI (*to* GUY) But it's gonna change, isn't it? All the time. It's not gonna be …

GUY Well, yes. But, I mean, one of the things about people is that they're incredibly adaptable. And you've seen that with Jonathan. He's adapted to a situation and, you know, he's on top of a lot of what's going on. And that won't *change* necessarily. So as things move on people get better at managing their own stuff. And if there comes a time when they *can't* do that then usually they can tell you what they need even if they can't do it. And I think that one of the essential things about being at home is seeing teamwork in a different kind of way. (*To* JONATHAN) And *you* are just as much part of the team as anybody else. And actually, if you come down to it your ability to monitor your own pain control – your ability to *know* if things are different to say the last time something happened – you're the only person who can tell us that. And if we give you the permission to actually act on those feelings and decisions then it makes life a lot easier actually to wind the whole sort of angst level down. And if you're dealing with something like pain, or any symptom like that, by and large if you anticipate the problems - or if you know what triggers it - then it may mean that you have to take something more seriously than usual. As long as you know what those are then it doesn't get out of control. It gets out of control when you're not quite sure what to do. (*To* VICKI) Or if you're worried about Jonathan and he's worried about you. And it's about being more relaxed. And that seems to be a daft thing to be saying if someone's got a fatal illness and they're planning to be at home and they're planning to die at home: "How can that be anything other than *awful*?" a lot of people will say. Well, it's usually quite the opposite.

VICKI Mmm … (*She speaks to camera*):

EVENTUALLY, I PULLED MYSELF TOGETHER before questioning Jonathan further about the tumours in his lungs. And when he drew an accurate diagram of them onto a blank sheet of paper, I was truly shocked by how much bigger they had grown since his last x-ray. I was also amazed by Jonathan's willingness to speak so openly about his private meeting with Julian. I took this as a positive sign that he is now ready to accept the final stage of his illness. Regardless, when he also told me that Julian was surprised he was not already experiencing major symptoms, I instantly knew Jonathan's current breathing situation was not good. And yet, for me, it was as though this final stage had arrived almost out of the blue. Because, undoubtedly, had he taken the suggested chemotherapy treatment back in January he would have looked - and felt - significantly worse than he has to date. He would also most likely have spent a large part of his time in hospital too. But apart from his dry, persistent cough and extremely pale complexion Jonathan has shown few visible signs of his disease. In fact, I felt strangely proud when he was recently weighed-in at the Oncology Clinic and had actually gained four pounds –

GUY (*to* JONATHAN) Because you're at home; you've got your stuff around you. You've got your videos; you've got your games; you're in a familiar environment; you know exactly what's there. You know what you like; you know what you *don't* like. So that actually takes *all* of that stuff away. And to be honest with you, sometimes it's more harm than good being in hospital 'cos we all worry and fuss around.

VICKI (*to* GUY) Yeah. Well, I fink the best solution would be to actually wise Jonathan up on the medication that he needs. 'Cos he's always known right from the beginning that he wants me an' him to deal with this together and with as little outside help. We know it's gotta be there but … with as little as possible.

GUY Well, it hasn't necessarily got to be there. I mean, you know, people *do* manage amazingly on their own. And we're here to make sure that this works for you. We're not here to make ourselves feel better. And we're not here to give ourselves a job to do. So, really, it's down to you to determine the level of support you get and what *kind* it is.

FLORA (*to* GUY) What's worked very well for us in the past is, armm, potential symptoms are pre-empted and, armm, a care plan is drawn-up and the medication is prescribed on an as and when needs basis, armm, and that is reassuring for *us* because we know that we can, armm, get his medication straight away … and also for the families and the kids as well.

TORI (*to* JONATHAN, *quickly*) What Flora's saying is that we can *anticipate* some of the issues. Anticipate, perhaps, problems that *might* happen so there can be a range of medication in the house. Do you see what I mean? So you feel more reassured that you've got something at home to help you with a pain, or … feeling sick, or something like that.

VICKI Well, yeah. I mean, *you* do this as a living. We've never done this before.

TORI (*nodding enthusiastically*) Exactly! Exactly. And you want to do it right.

JONATHAN (*to* TORI) So you're gonna go on past experiences – on what you've seen before – an' you're gonna give us medication for that?

TORI On what you *tell* us. On what you tell us. You're the best guide.

JONATHAN 'Cos I don't know what's gonna happen. I don't know *how* I'm gonna feel, do I?

TORI No. But you'll *know* when you feel a bit more breathless. And you'll *know* when you're a bit more tired or whenever there's any pain and things like that.

GUY (*to* JONATHAN) I mean, the truth is that, you know, we can *guess* what's gonna happen.

JONATHAN Yeah. That's what I mean.

GUY And we've probably got a fifty-fifty chance of being right if not less. And the way *you* handle what happens – and the way things develop – we deal with as they come along. You know, we should have you effectively pain free. (*Pause*) And that's what we need to aim for. Alright? And there are lots and lots of medications. Lots of tricks that we can put together to make that easier for you and give you various options.

JONATHAN Medications?

GUY Yeah. And, you know, *tailoring* it to your requirements is really down to you. I mean, you have to experiment with every individual patient as to what combinations of things are the best. And then, relatively quickly you'll be on top of that and you'll know how to do it for yourself. And you'll do it far better than we can because you'll know how to monitor yourself. Breathlessness. Feeling tired. All those kinds of things. Or other symptoms: you might feel sick – that's another symptom.

JONATHAN Cough.

GUY Coughing – that's another thing. So that's the management side. And then there's the *coping* side which is slightly different. (*Pause*) You know, looking from the outside *we* think something's an issue and it isn't actually. And so, you've got to have the permission and the authority to say, "Well, actually, no. I'm fine here. Just clear off!" You know? "I don't wanna see you today! I've got other things to do. I've got other people to see. You're not coming in the afternoon- I'm watching a movie!" (JONATHAN *half laughs*) So it's that kind of thing.

FLORA (*to* JONATHAN) And I think also, armm, we should feel comfortable, you know, if you're not happy with something that *we're* doing and vice versa, you know, we should be able to communicate honestly with each other. I think that's really important. Honesty and communication.

VICKI (*to* FLORA) What? On a twenty-four hour basis? 'Cos I'm worried: you work nine to four an' then suddenly after four o/clock it's down to me. And like *you* said (*she turns to* GUY) summinks *bound* to happen when I can't get hold of someone. And that scares me.

FLORA (*slowly*) Yeah, armm, we will provide a twenty-four hour service, armm, but not right at the beginning, armm … but we'll always make sure that there's somebody that, armm, there's always someone …

ROB (*to* FLORA) The Bexley team works out of hours, doesn't it?

TORI (*to* VICKI) And that's the *teamwork* Guy was alluding to. Now, we're *thinking* that probably Greenwich and Bexley provide a twenty-four hour service so *they* can take over when Dora's team aren't there. Does that make sense? Now if they don't that will be Guy's team. Does that make sense? So there'll be a way, like Guy says, of plugging the gaps so there is a twenty-four …

VICKI (*leaning forward in her seat and looking directly into* JONATHAN*'s large, hazel eyes*) Would you consider talking to someone from the hospice now? We did talk about it and you absolutely threw it out the window but in the circumstances, as they're professionally able to help us, would you *consider* … Not to actually *go* there or anyfing like that but just to …

JONATHAN Talk to them?

VICKI More supporting *me* … to be able to help *you* 'cos I feel …

JONATHAN You're talking about mentally being able to cope, aren't yer?

TORI (*quickly*) No darling. We're talking about two different things.

VICKI *Physically* being able to cope with being up all night an' day; trying to be on call for you. It's really, I mean, as it stands now I'm up 'til three in the morning waiting to see if you need me to take you to the hospital. It's gonna get worse …

GUY Hold on! Do you stay up 'til three o/clock in the morning worrying about him?

VICKI I do, yeah.

GUY Why?

VICKI 'Cos of the breathing trouble that he had the other night. And now I'm worried that it's gonna happen again an' I might go into such a deep …

GUY (*to* JONATHAN) What happened then?

JONATHAN Well, at three o/clock in the morning I couldn't breathe properly so I had to go to the hospital.

GUY (*rubbing his round chin whilst lightly nodding*) Right. Right.

VICKI And I have to get up with my uvver children and that means I've only had about three or four hours sleep, which I can cope on but that's gonna get worse and I'm worried that I can't relax at all knowing… 'Cos it's me he wants to be there but I'm gonna need breaks from the …

GUY No. No. No. That's fine.

(*Together*)

VICKI Sitting there and being on call.

GUY (*to* JONATHAN) How often have you had breathing problems like that?

JONATHAN Oh, only for about a week. That was the worst one though.

GUY And what? It came on over a few hours or came on quite suddenly or … ?

JONATHAN It came on *fairly* suddenly, yeah. Over a few hours. It started at about midnight.

GUY (*to* TORI) Was it an asthmatic problem?

TORI (*softly*) No. No.

JONATHAN It wasn't like I stopped breathing. It was just *difficulty* breathing, like … painful.

GUY Like taking a deep breath, or … ?

JONATHAN Yeah. Very painful. That type of difficulty, yeah.

VICKI (*to* GUY) This is what's prompted me to contact Flora and Tori.

TORI (*to* JONATHAN, *quickly*) And this is why, Jonathan, when I spoke to you this morning and you told me you've got your cough, didn't you? (JONATHAN *nods*) You've got your pain that you're controlling with your codeine and paracetamol but you're taking those incredibly regularly, aren't you?

JONATHAN Yeah.

TORI So you've got your cough; breathlessness every now and then; temperatures, which are probably to do with the disease that you have; (*she points to his chest*) and you've got your pain here, which is why it's *really* good that Guy's here as well because we can talk about these things and try and sort them out for you *today* because I'm not quite sure you're completely pain-free, are you? Even taking all those painkillers.

JONATHAN No. I'm not.

TORI (*quickly*) And this is what we mean about the fact that if you *tell* us things then we can help you with them. And when you said earlier *What, to help you mentally*? You know. You don't have to have that if you don't want to but what mum's talking about is whether you'd be happy for us to get in touch with someone at Greenwich and Bexley to help on *these* sort of issues: if you did have some breathlessness in the middle of the night. The other side we can come to in a minute.

JONATHAN (*slightly bewildered*) Yeah. Well, I would need help wouldn't I?

TORI Yeah. Exactly! But because mum respects you, darling, she wants your permission to do that. She wouldn't dream of just saying "go and refer him to so and so" without asking your permission. But it's all difficult 'cos it's all part of a process and that can be hard 'cos hospices are only associated with one thing and that can make it a little bit like …

GUY (*to* TORI) Sorry. Can I be boring and try to get a handle on what's going on here? (*To* JONATHAN) The first time that you got breathing problems was a few days ago? Or last week? Or something like that? And that was just generally bothering you on and off? Or regular? Or worse, or … How did it go?

JONATHAN What? Ever since I got it and ever since I went to hospital about it?

GUY Mmm …

JONATHAN Well, it was kinda always there but it was difficulty in breathing. Every time I took a breath in there was pain in my chest and every time I breathed out it was pain. An' around the back as well.

VICKI (*to* GUY) *And* when he lies down.

GUY (*to* JONATHAN) So pain was the issue *not* the breathing?

JONATHAN Yeah.

VICKI (*to* GUY) *And* the breathing. He felt he needed oxygen. That's what he felt he needed.

GUY Yeah. (*To* JONATHAN) Did you get wound-up when all this was going on?

JONATHAN Did I get what?

GUY Did it wind you up? Make you anxious?

JONATHAN Yeah. That's why I called mum in and asked her to take me to the hospital.

GUY Yeah. Sure. I understand. Okay. Right. Right. And once the pain was controlled did the breathlessness go away?

JONATHAN The pain wasn't really controlled. The paracetamols wasn't really working, nor was the codeine. But that's cos I wasn't taking them so regularly as I am now. An' now the pain is …

GUY Much better?

JONATHAN Slightly. Yeah.

GUY (*softly*) Okay. I mean, that's a very manageable thing. We can explain to you and show you how to do that. And that is actually the kind of thing that you can deal with over the telephone if things are difficult or problematical. We just have a conversation on the 'phone.

VICKI Yeah?

GUY Or the Bexley team can have conversation on the phone. If you *do* need to come into hospital well … we just fix it, you know? It's not a problem.

VICKI (*to* GUY) The problem I've also got wiv Jonathan is that he does leave fings to the last minute too, which worries me when the responsibility is on my shoulders and I'm the only one in the house to deal wiv it. He *will not* complain! He didn't complain until half past twelve at night *then* I found out he was having problems a lot earlier: hours and hours earlier! And if the problems – his symptoms – are gonna get worse and he's not telling *me* what's going on … I can't stand by an' watch summink … you know? It's gonna happen too quick for him … an' I need to be in control. (*She speaks to camera*):

JONATHAN ATTEMPTED TO GO OUT with his friends last Wednesday evening. But he soon returned home due to another severe leg cramp. And in all his frustration, he stormed up the stairs and straight into his bedroom the instant I opened the front door.

"Leave me alone!" he yelled, each time I offered my assistance.

But I didn't leave him. Instead, like a constant shadow I hovered on the landing outside Jonathan's bedroom door listening to him huff and puff his way through the usual leg exercises that were now proving to be useless. Worried and concerned, I timidly offered to help my stubborn son several more times but he still rejected my assistance. All I could do was weep in sheer frustration as I anxiously paced up and down the cramped landing that is filled with an over-flowing bookcase; an electric radiator; a blue swivel chair; a red bean bag; and a big television set on which the boys play their computer games. Time tiptoed alongside me. Approximately one hour passed. Then, suddenly, Jonathan's bedroom door flew open. Appearing exhausted, he collapsed inside the open doorway. I raced towards him. Desperate to rid him of his debilitating pain, I began to massage his withered left leg. Jonathan's flushed face grew even hotter. His furrowed brow glistened. Regardless, I continued to massage his painful limb in an attempt to ease his excruciating pain. But Jonathan still writhed in agony. I wept. Then I suddenly thought to give him a muscle relaxant. But, sadly, that failed us too. In total despair, I silently prayed for some divine intervention to miraculously release my precious boy from his acute suffering. More hours passed. Eventually, Jonathan allowed Richard to take over from me whilst I attempted to contact a paediatrician at our local hospital. But, to my horror, there were none on duty. Frantically, I searched through Jonathan's medical notes in the hope that the Cancer Unit could help us. But because he has not attended the Unit for some time I could not find them. Regardless, I blindly telephoned the switchboard operator at the central London hospital and explained our dilemma. I was eventually connected to a palliative care nurse named Margaret who calmly advised me to give Jonathan a painkiller. Another hour passed. Jonathan's strength was now almost fully depleted, but he still writhed in agony. I telephoned Margaret once more. And when she advised me to give him another painkiller *plus* another muscle relaxant, I finally sighed with relief as I watched my distressed son slip into a deep, involuntary sleep.

It was near 4 a.m. before Richard and I went to bed that evening. And I cannot say which of us was the most exhausted! But I can say that I will never forget the severe suffering Jonathan endured on that agonising night. I can also say that I will never forget the huge sense of failure I felt at being unable to help my cherished son in his hour of need. Anyhow, I telephoned both Flora and Simon from the Greenwich and Bexley Hospice the instant I awoke the next morning and they both visited us later that same day. Thankfully, Jonathan's medication has now been changed. And I pray his new prescription will help should we ever find ourselves in a similar situation. Incidentally, Jonathan's home tutor, Sally, also paid us an unexpected visit on that same day. She wanted to tell Jonathan that she has nominated him to receive recognition at the 'Do the Right Thing' awards ceremony that is to be held at our local town hall on the 6th June. Naturally, my proud son beamed with pride when Sally told him that she thought him remarkable for the way in which he has coped with his academic work whilst being ill. However, to date, Jonathan has refused to commit to the evening mainly because he does not know how he will feel on the night and also because he may not even receive a prize. Nevertheless, Sally reassured him that he can change his mind at any time -

GUY (*to* JONATHAN) What's the reason you don't tell your mum?

JONATHAN Well, the first reason is 'cos I fink it might go away an' it might be unnecessary worry.

GUY Yep, which is fair.

JONATHAN Yeah. And, er, well that's both reasons really: unnecessary worry an' it might go away. So I feel … (*very softly*) just leave it then. Just let it go. Keep it to myself. (*Pause*) But I *did* tell her eventually.

VICKI (*to* GUY) But then there was a panic and I wanna avoid the panic!

GUY Yeah. I think if we *know* the way Jonathan is communicating about his symptoms, or whatever it is, then you say: "Okay. We need to get an ambulance." And that's the sum total of it rather than getting into a complete worry about things. So I think if we look at helping the two of you to *monitor* how the symptoms are going, or whether something's changing over a period of time, and then say: "Well, okay. If it's getting to this place …" Let's take a hypothetical: Let's say we re-ran the twelve-thirty breathlessness problem again, okay? Let's say Jonathan (*he turns to* JONATHAN) probably about eight or nine or ten o/clock in the evening you started to feel a bit funny?

JONATHAN (*softly*) That's right, yeah.

GUY That would be a time to say: "Just not feeling too clever." And then, instead of worrying about it saying: "Okay, well let's see what it's feeling like in two hours, or an hour's time." Take your painkillers – 'cos that would be the time to take your painkillers – then at eight or nine o/clock in the evening, if the pain's *not* under control or if you're feeling more breathlessness after say two hours, *then* make a phone call. And then, based on that phone call it's either "Straight in" *or* "Let's make an adjustment to the pain control. Let's review it again in an hour. There's no change in an hour: you're in!" So what you've got is a controlled process over a four or five hour period and you're not all sitting on the edge of the bed worrying and waiting 'til three o/clock 'cos actually you probably should have been admitted at about one rather than getting to three. Do you follow me? That's just an example of a different way of managing the problem. The problem is still there. The problem needs an admission but actually the *anxiety* around it is much less.

VICKI (*Quickly*) The problem that actually arose more than anyfing was … I actually *knew* - when I was taking him to the hospital at three in the morning - that I was gonna have to take him. I *knew*. The problem arose with *when* he would let me take him. That was the problem.

JONATHAN (*to* VICKI, *defensively*) The problem is at three o/clock in the morning you're always reluctant to get up and go to hospital.

It's not the kinda thing you wanna do that early in the morning.

(*Together*)

VICKI As soon as you told me at half-twelve I thought …

"Right. I'm gonna have to take you to the hospital!" (*To* GUY) But it was waiting until he would say to me: "Right. It's bad now." I *knew* I should have taken him earlier but he wouldn't let me. So …

GUY (*to* JONATHAN) But you're gonna negotiate that, aren't you? ''Cos you're not gonna make that mistake again, are you? So next time, if it's eight o/clock then by eleven, half-eleven, you've made a decision …

JONATHAN Straight away.

GUY And then deal with it.

TORI (*quickly*) And it may mean that you don't need to go into hospital, Jonathan, if you do the steps that Guy was telling you about.

Do you see what I mean?

(*Together*)

JONATHAN I know. That's what I'm thinking.

TORI 'Cos you know you hate hospitals!

GUY See? It sounds to me – just listening to the breathlessness story – that actually the problem was pain control. And that if we got the pain under control then you would have got to the stage when you could take a breath in. 'Cos there's a particular kind of breathlessness that's associated with anxiety and the sense is that you can't get a big enough breath in. Is that what you were?

JONATHAN Yeah.

GUY Right. Okay. So that's an anxiety based breathlessness rather than a problem with the lungs kind of breathlessness. I can't get a breath in and the reason for that is if I take a breath I get pain. I don't want to take a breath for the pain but I want to take a breath! (JONATHAN *laughs*) And so you get into this cycle. And actually, that was all to do with pain control.

JONATHAN 'Cos as soon as it goes away you can breathe!

VICKI He's asthmatic as well which caused a bit of confusion.

GUY Sure. (*To* JONATHAN) But *you* know the difference. That breathlessness wasn't asthmatic breathlessness, right? *You* know the difference?

JONATHAN No. Definitely.

GUY (*to* VICKI) Right. So he knows the difference.

NICKI But he didn't tell *me* that!

GUY No. I know. But he's telling you now.

VICKI That's my point.

GUY He's telling you now, okay? (*To* JONATHAN) So I think a lot of the stuff is around making sure we're communicating accurately.

VICKI Mmm …(*Pause*) I think Jonathan's gotta learn …

GUY (*pointing at* JONATHAN) But he's got pain and discomfort at the moment from the way he's moving around. (*To* JONATHAN) Is that right?

JONATHAN Mmm.

GUY So we may need to look at …

VICKI (*to* GUY) He's got to allow *me* to look for outside help so that

I can then help him 'cos he hasn't been letting me do that.

GUY Yeah. And you've got to allow *him* to call the shots.

VICKI Yeah. If he wants to be nursed at home and not in hospital I've *got* to get some support from outside, which he's been reluctant for me to do up to now.

TORI (*to* VICKI, *quickly*) But what Jonathan is also saying is that he's not ready to give-up control either.

JONATHAN No.

(*Together*)

VICKI No.

TORI (*to* JONATHAN) And *you* wanna call the shots. But you *can* call the shots if mum's got a bit more support! Does that seem fair?

JONATHAN (*submissively*) I know. I know. That's fair.

GUY (*to* JONATHAN) Do I just need to talk to you about this, erm, chest pain – discomfort – you're experiencing now? Do you need to talk about that?

JONATHAN (*shuffling in his seat and softly mumbling to himself*) I don't know what …

GUY You're uncomfortable though, aren't you?

JONATHAN (*examining his seat*) Perhaps it's the way I'm sitting.

GUY (*disbelievingly*) Is it?

TORI You *have* got pain though, haven't you?

(JONATHAN *shifts his body to his extreme right and fumbles beneath his seat. Presently, he produces his empty bottle of natural spring water that he has been unwittingly sitting on. He grins widely at both* GUY *and* TORI.)

GUY Oh, right! He's sitting on a bottle!

(*The whole room instantly fills with laughter.*)

JONATHAN (*Still smiling*) Sorry mates. I need to use the loo.

(*There is a long pause as* JONATHAN *exits the room. And* VICKI *observes the big beech-wood door as it slowly closes behind him. She speaks to camera.*):

AFTER MUCH DISCUSSION, JONATHAN AND I decided not to attend the standard appointment that was automatically arranged for us to see a lung specialist. In fact, to our surprise, it is usual hospital practice to offer all patients like Jonathan an operation that involves 'gluing' the lungs back onto the chest cavity in order to prevent them from collapsing too quickly. But Jonathan and I both think this extreme operation sounds too risky for our liking. And, most importantly, it will not prevent his tumours from growing any faster. And so we have declined the operation on the grounds that this type of major surgery will only intensify Jonathan's physical suffering without making a scrap of difference to his condition.

SCENE TWO

VICKI (*casually, to* GUY, TORI, *and* FLORA *whilst* JONATHAN *is still out of the room.*) They're anti-inflammatory. (*She touches her left arm and shoulder.*) They will probably take the pressure off the nerve that's causing the pain down his arm. But 'cos his brother's just been diagnosed with Crohns disease and *he's* on steroids and been told they make you chubby and they make you spotty … he's vain! He's fifteen and he's vain! And he doesn't wanna be spotty and he doesn't wanna get fat! (*She speaks to camera*):

THEY SAY IT NEVER RAINS but it pours. And now I can confirm this old adage to be true since Richard was recently diagnosed with Crohns disease. Admittedly, I noticed he was looking unwell for some time but simply bought him some multi-vitamins and thought no more of it. However, only a few weeks passed before I was abruptly awoken by a loud crashing noise coming from somewhere downstairs. But due to extreme tiredness I shamefully ignored it and soon drifted back into a deep sleep. Anyway, only minutes passed before the loud crashing noise woke me once more. This time it was much louder. My sleepy mind switched into overdrive. My heart quickened. And yet I had no time to make sense out of the noisy commotion that was now racing up the stairs in an extremely clumsy manner. Fear engulfed me. In terror, my entire body froze when my bedroom door suddenly flew open. It took a few moments for my startled eyes to recognise Richard who - in his boxer shorts – was doubled over inside the open doorway. His pale frame appeared unusually thin and bony. His strenuous breathing alarmed me further. I almost screamed but before I could make a sound Richard had stumbled to the side of my bed:

"Mum. I'm *really* ill." He wheezed, laboriously.

Then, like a pile of sticks, he collapsed on top of me. I was stunned. Desperately trying to free myself from beneath his bony weight, I soon panicked again when I caught sight of the bright-red blood that saturated his entire lower body. Richard awoke. And in a dazed state, he blindly ran out of my bedroom before collapsing, once again, onto the landing floor. My confused mind struggled to make sense out of what was happening. In truth, I believed my eldest son was dying. Grabbing a pillow off my blood-stained bed, I dashed onto the landing and fell to my knees beside Richard. Gently placing the warm pillow beneath his pale head, I cradled him in my shaky arms. His vacant eyes stared back at me from inside his deathly grey complexion. His capsized chest groaned loudly. He was clearly in shock. And so was I. Especially when I caught sight of the fresh clumps of bright-red blood that were now forming into a small pool around us. I finally screamed very loudly. And, within seconds, Jonathan was kneeling close beside me. Strangely, I noticed he was fully clothed and wearing his prosthesis.

"Stay in your room!" I screeched to Daniel and Rosie, when I saw their bedroom door handle slowly turn. "Oh, God! I think he's dying!" I whispered to Jonathan.

"Ricky! Don't sleep!" Jonathan repeatedly commanded.

But dazed Richard continued to drift in and out of consciousness. In total despair, Jonathan shouted at me:

"Mum! Ring for an ambulance! Be quick! Ring for it now!"

Nervously sitting on the top step of our bloody stairwell, I tearfully relayed our dilemma to the calm voice on the other end of the telephone line. Meanwhile, Jonathan continued ordering Richard not to sleep until an ambulance arrived.

Thankfully, Richard's symptoms are now under control. But it certainly was a difficult week for everyone. Indeed, trying to divide my time equally between both Richard in hospital and Jonathan at home was extremely testing to say the least -

GUY (*to* VICKI) Do you think we need to get him to come-up to the clinic to see me? Would that be helpful? And we'll sit down and do a proper symptom review. So why don't we arrange it for Friday – if you ring through to say that you're here then I can sit down and do a proper analyse of what drugs he's on. And if he doesn't play by the rules and he gets symptoms then that's his problem.

TORI (*to* VICKI, *quickly*) But it's not because we'll also support you with that. But what Guy's talking like that for is so that Jonathan knows that … At the moment the deal is Jonathan wants to take control. But if he doesn't play the game …

GUY (*to* VICKI) Yeah. I'm gonna have to tell you that I think this is a bloke thing.

TORI And he's *always* been like that!

VICKI (*to* GUY) Yeah. *And* it's a teenage fing.

TORI Yep!

GUY 'Course it is.

VICKI It's like: "Mum can't tell me what to do twenty-four hours a day!" (*Incidentally*) And we *are* together twenty-four hours a day.

TORI (*quickly*) And also, he feels very exposed which Guy *doesn't* know about. He's been very exposed to other young people dying. You know, he reminds us about Claire. He saw Fran too. He's been very exposed to that. So on the one hand, although he's wanting to be in control all these things are signals to what he saw happening to other people as well. You know, so he's protecting himself slightly there as well.

VICKI Definitely. And the worst scenario for Jonathan is that he will end-up in so much pain; he's in hospital; and that's where he's gonna stay!

TORI (*vigorously shaking her head*) And that's *not* gonna happen.

GUY (*reassuringly*) No. That won't happen.

TORI And you're *not* on your own, Vicki.

VICKI 'Cos that's what he doesn't want.

GUY I look after enough dying people to know the patients it's gonna work with and the patients it isn't gonna work with. And it's gonna work with him. It'll be alright. And you have to accept the fact that he is still who he is. And so it's getting a balance between *that* as well as managing the illness.

TORI (*quickly*) And what he's also saying though, Vicki, is although the idea of the hospice seems lovely to all of us – going somewhere that's really tranquil and peaceful – to Jonathan that's not his life experience. And actually what he's saying, despite the fact he might moan about it, is he wants to be at home as part of his family.

GUY (*quietly*) He's going to come back in.

(*There is a long pause. And as* JONATHAN *politely re-enters the room,* VICKI *observes the big beech-wood door as it slowly closes behind him.*)

GUY (*hesitantly, to* VICKI) We're about there, aren't we?

VICKI (*very tiredly*) Okay then. Fanks. (*To* JONATHAN, *humorously*) Sorted?

TORI (*laughingly*) He doesn't want to discuss where he's been, do you Jonathan?

GUY (*lightly*) No. We won't talk about that. (*To* JONATHAN) So you're gonna be up for some radiotherapy tomorrow?

JONATHAN Well … hopefully.

GUY So shall we plan to sit down with all your drug lists …

JONATHAN (*positively*) Yeah. That will be good.

GUY And I want to talk to you properly about the pain and how we can manage that. Okay? So we'll go over that in detail. Alright?

JONATHAN Yeah. That would be helpful that would.

GUY But I was saying to your mum: I think we're well ahead of the game on this and it's gonna be fine. It really is.

JONATHAN Alright. Cheers.

FLORA (*to* GUY, *timidly*) Armm, would you like me to speak to Greenwich and Bexley? I'll put some feelers out.

GUY If you have a word with them and then I'll speak to them as necessary. (*He looks at* JONATHAN) We're nowhere *near* having to have people going in all the time to you and all this kind of stuff. So I think I'd rather get you kind of educated on how to deal with your symptoms …

JONATHAN By myself.

GUY By yourself. And then we can take it from there.

TORI As a partnership with your mum.

JONATHAN (*positively*) Yeah. I was gonna 'ave that. Yeah.

TORI Good! (*Teasingly, in a mock cockney accent*) I'm glad yer gonna 'ave that!

(*Everybody laughs.* JONATHAN *smiles at* VICKI *as he affectionately taps her shoulder.*)

GUY Excellent! Good! We're done now. That's a wrap!

(GUY *rises from his seat. He walks briskly towards the door and speaks with* CAROLINE *about further filming before he exits the room.*)

SCENE THREE

There is a long pause. Everyone inside the room becomes more relaxed. CAROLINE, JACK, *and* MAX, *who are still standing by the door, remain perfectly silent. In order to be closer to* JONATHAN, TORI *moves into* GUY's *vacant chair. Finally,* FLORA *fully reclines into her seat. Whilst* VICKI – *in a sleepy and tired manner -slouches across the arm of the small, navy sofa. (She speaks to camera)*:

TORI WAS THE FIRST PERSON we met when we arrived at the Oncology Clinic on that cold and dreary Monday morning back in January, 2000. Naturally, as a family, we had a tough time getting through the Christmas festivities knowing that Jonathan was seriously ill. And, of course, we had absolutely no idea what to expect from our first visit to such an unfamiliar place. But, thankfully, Tori was there to greet us. Her warm, approachable manner helped to put us at ease as we waited to see Doctor Julian. She also had extensive medical knowledge and did her utmost to answer our countless questions. She even accompanied us to Jonathan's consultation so that we felt supported. Then she gave us a preliminary tour of the Cancer Unit so that we could accustom ourselves with the ward prior to Jonathan commencing treatment. However, apart from Tori's professional expertise and obvious kindness, I mostly appreciate the way in which she has always treated us with total respect. Fortunately for us, Tori stayed at the Cancer Unit long enough to see Jonathan through his gruelling chemotherapy treatment and amputation before taking some maternity leave. And, to our delight, when we returned to Julian's clinic exactly one year later for Jonathan's routine check-up Tori was, once again, there to greet us. Her fortifying presence on that fateful day back in January - when we were unexpectedly told that Jonathan had relapsed in his lungs - will never be forgotten. Indeed, that particular appointment will always remain the most memorable simply because the goal posts determining my cherished son's future suddenly shifted.

Within moments of meeting Julian our intense and over-riding desire for Jonathan to be given the all-clear was cruelly snatched away from us. Only to be replaced with the stark realisation of knowing that my brave and fearless son was no longer fighting for his life but only for a dignified death –

TORI (*very softly*) Jonathan and Vicki?

(JONATHAN *and* VICKI *look at* TORI. *Instinctively,* VICKI *shuffles along the sofa in order to be closer to* JONATHAN. *The trio form a closed circle.*) I'm just being very aware for both of you that some of the stuff we spoke about seems so bad. (TORI *lightly touches* VICKI'*s arm in a supportive manner.*) I'm not gonna say for a minute that any of it has helped. He's your boy. If we could give you more than this you're still gonna sit there worrying.

VICKI But I can only work in a direct way, Tori. I can't …

TORI (*quickly*) Exactly! (*She looks at* JONATHAN) And *he* knows you well enough. If you suddenly said: "Oh, Jonathan. Do what you want darling." He'd be thinking "What the *hell* is wrong with my mum!" (JONATHAN *grins widely*) You've still got to be you and he's *always* gonna be him.

VICKI He wants me to be the main nurse in all this so I've gotta be practical too, haven't I?

TORI (*to* JONATHAN) But that's true what I've just said: she's always gonna be her and you're gonna be you. Yep? (JONATHAN *softly nods in agreement.*) But where there just has to be a little bit of movement, which is what Guy has said, is for her to allow you to be you … 'cos she's gonna want to get this right, darling.

JONATHAN I know. I know.

TORI And it's *so* difficult to talk about, I know. But you just need to …

JONATHAN I *try* not to push her away too much.

TORI Yeah. But that's all very complex. (*Then humorously*) With you … the way you are!

(VICKI *laughs aloud.*)

JONATHAN (*to* VICKI, *humorously*) Huh! What's *that* look for?

TORI No, but also Jonathan – the way you are – it's all so complicated 'cos you wanna protect her and you don't want to worry her and she doesn't want to dump on you.

JONATHAN Right.

TORI (*quickly*) And those are the things when you said about: "Oh, the hospice! For the mental stuff!" I know what you mean by that. It's like, you know, people have this image that you've got to be all prepared properly. What you're going through is *horrible*. You know, we sit here chatting and we've all been laughing with Guy and it's like: "What are they *really* talking about?" (JONATHAN *half laughs*) And we're talking about you dying! Do you know what I mean? And look at your mum. She looks great today. I'd probably be …

VICKI (*defensively*) Yeah. But you don't see what goes on at home, do you?

TORI No. That's what I'm saying. And we appreciate that. It's *awful*. (*To* JONATHAN) And you sit there and you make it so easy for us because you protect all of us. But we do *know* that it's tough. And it's hard. (JONATHAN *softly agrees*) And I wouldn't sit here saying: "Jonathan. I think you're feeling this and I think you're feeling that." 'Cos that would be an insult to you.

JONATHAN Yeah.

TORI And you'd tell me to get lost! But there might come a time when you *need* to talk. And mum's right in so much that because you protect her you might not want to tell her. And that's when there'll be a group of people around. And you'll choose the right time.

JONATHAN I know I will.

TORI Or you might not want to. And that's perfectly right too 'cos you'll do it Jonathan's way. Just like you've done it from the very first day you were diagnosed. Haven't you?

(*Once again,* VICKI *laughs aloud whilst* JONATHAN *grins widely. There is a long, reflective pause. And as the two women gaze at* JONATHAN *in a warm and affectionate manner, he visibly ponders over* TORI*'s insightful words.*)

JONATHAN (*still smiling*) Jonathan's way …

TORI Yeah. Jonathan's way!

(*Long pause*)

FLORA (*almost inaudibly*) And you're the main player in this team, Jonathan.

TORI (*quickly*) You *are* the main player but we've also got to look out for her too.

(*Once again,* TORI *lightly touches* VICKI*'s arm.*)

JONATHAN (*submissively*) I know. I know.

TORI (*very seriously*) And I think meeting Guy tomorrow will be really good.

JONATHAN So we've got a plan for fings.

TORI Yep! And then, actually, although that's hard then *you're* back in control again. Does that make sense?

JONATHAN Yeah. Yeah. That'll take away a lot of uncertainty when it actually … I get in pain.

TORI Exactly!

VICKI (*to* JONATHAN, *kindly*) Is that why you get really cross wiv me 'cos I try to control the tablets an' … yer know, when your meant to take 'em an' stuff? 'Cos it makes you feel like you're losing some sort of control?

JONATHAN (*lightly scratching his head*) I dunno. I s'pose … in a way. But, obviously, I wouldn't take the tablets if I didn't wanna. So …

(*Pause*)

VICKI (*tiredly rubbing her forehead*) Well … I'll trust you then.

TORI (*to* JONATHAN, *quickly*) Also, you've got a right to be angry! You know, as much as you've sat here laughing and joking with us all I'd be furious if I was you, Jonathan. Do you know what I mean? (JONATHAN *mutters something inaudible beneath his breath.*) On the other hand, you try to make it so easy for all of us. But it *is* unfair! And it's horrible. Do you know what I mean? It's like the way your mum looks. It's all very well. And we've talked. You know: "Talked about that. Got to get this right. And I want to do this …" And it's alright while you're mum's talking – and she looks great today – but we know at home she must break her heart and get upset. (*There is another long pause. An extremely sad and unusually solemn expression suddenly washes over* JONATHAN*'s handsome young face. He quickly averts* *his large, hazel eyes towards the tiny sash window behind him.*) Do you know what I mean? So we *know* there's another side to it. It's not just how you're presenting here today.

JONATHAN (*very softly*) I know.

VICKI You don't judge a book by its cover, do you?

TORI Exactly! And it's fatal if you do! You *mustn't*. We *know* there's another side.

VICKI (*quietly*) There is.

TORI (*to* JONATHAN, *quickly*) And that's why it's all very well us wanting to listen to you, and if we all sat there and said: "Ahh, poor Jonathan. He should be allowed to do what he likes." (*She half laughs*) Meanwhile, you've got mum at home tearing her hair out! (*She nods at* VICKI) Which is why the word 'teamwork' is so important. (*Sincerely, but still smiling*) And you're a good double act. And you've got those other people at home that love you as well, haven't you?

(*Pause*)

VICKI (*to* JONATHAN) So you don't mind me calling outside help when I need it?

JONATHAN (*almost enthusiastically*) No. 'Course I don't. (*Then defensively to* TORI, *who is playfully smiling at him in disbelief.*) No. I don't actually.

TORI Alright. And Guy's very blunt. He's very honest. He's probably as blunt and honest as you are actually. You've probably met your match! (JONATHAN *laughs aloud.*) *And* he doesn't waffle. 'Cos you don't like waffle, do you?

VICKI (*humorously*) And he's a bloke, Jonny!

TORI (*quickly*) And he's a bloke! (*Still playfully and in a highly exaggerated south London accent*) Not annuver woman to nag yer! (*The trio instantly laugh in unison.*) (*Pause*) Alright?

JONATHAN (*softly*) Yeah. I'm alright.

VICKI Fair enough. Thanks Tori. Thanks Flora.

FLORA (*very quietly*) Oh, that's alright.

(*Pause.* VICKI *speaks to camera*):

FLORA SURPRISED US WITH AN unexpected visit late last Friday afternoon. Standing inside our front doorway, I watched her trundle down the stony footpath carrying two small cylinders of oxygen in each hand. In silence, Jonathan stood close behind me.

"I've brought you these in case you have another emergency over the weekend," Flora puffed, when she eventually reached us.

Naturally, I thanked Flora for her kindness. But Jonathan was completely mortified by her "thoughtlessness" and total lack of discretion.

"I *hope* no-one saw her!" He angrily twitched, as Flora tottered back up the footpath. Then Jonathan searched up and down the crescent in an agitated manner to ensure that no-one was looking in our direction.

"Calm down, Jonathan! Flora was only being helpful." I told him, firmly.

"Yeah, well. She could've covered 'em wiv summink! I don't want ev'ryone knowing my business, do I?" He quickly retorted, in an unusually blunt manner.

I said no more. Instead, I took the heavy cylinders from Jonathan and carried them into our back room, which is mostly filled with garden equipment; lots of coats; and half-dried laundry. Jonathan trundled close behind me.

"Quick! Cover 'em wiv coats! I don't want 'em seen!" He ordered.

And although I desperately wanted to discuss Jonathan's current breathing difficulties, I soon surmised that this was not the right moment. Anyhow, it was early evening before Jonathan finally re-joined me inside our kitchen. He was still clearly anxious. Unflustered, I continued humming along to my favourite Costello soundtrack whilst preparing the evening meal. Jonathan sat quietly at the kitchen table.

"Mum. D'ya fink I'm well enough to go out with my friends?" He eventually asked.

I thought very long and carefully before I replied:

"Well … only you can be the judge of that one, babes. You're the only one who knows *exactly* how you feel."

My complete lack of authority only vexed Jonathan further.

"But I *really* need to see my mates!" He desperately cried.

I joined him at the table.

"Of course, I understand that, Jonny. I *really* do. But be truthful with yourself. How's yer breathing?"

"Well …" Jonathan sighed, heavily. "I *fink* it's alright. I just don't know if …"

He grew more anxious. His left knee bounced up and down in

a rapid manner. And when his large, hazel eyes overflowed with tears he jumped to his feet and began to pace up and down the kitchen floor like a caged lion. I almost crumbled. Yet I calmly said:

"Jon. I can't decide for you. But if you stay local then at least … ."

And with that, Jonathan sprang out of the kitchen and straight out of the front door. I raced to the front-room window. Through crisp-white netting, I observed the cautious manner in which my determined son greeted his much loved friends. However, when I saw the enormous effort he needed to make in order to keep up with them, I finally wept. Anyhow, within minutes, Jonathan's good friend, Dean, telephoned to inform me that he had collapsed in a nearby street. I dashed to my car. And with Dean's kind assistance, Jonathan was soon home again. But, in truth, I have never seen my proud and fearless son look quite as sad, or despondent, as he did on that night. Indeed, he endured another severe leg cramp that lasted several hours. He struggled with his laborious breathing too. And yet, it is his weak and feeble voice insisting to his friends that they must go on without him that has stayed in the forefront of my mind. Because only I know the true depth of that invisible pain and, of all things, how it hurts Jonathan the most.

Scene closes to 'Brave New World'
sung by Richard Ashcroft.

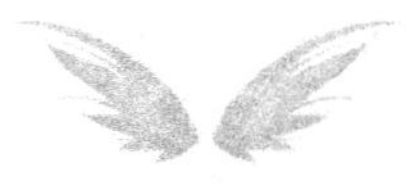

ACT FOUR

In Dreams

Characters

JONATHAN, attempting to grow a full moustache and goatee beard, is noticeably more breathless than in previous scenes. Frequently inhaling short, sharp breathes his soft speech is much slower and less fluent. His pale complexion appears slightly jaundiced. He is thinner too. And yet, his resolution to remain in strict control of his own physical (and spiritual) destiny remains unaltered.

CAROLINE, despite appearing a lot more at ease than in Act One, is obviously cautious about meeting with JONATHAN for the last time. Her hesitant speech is less formal than in previous scenes. She sounds lighter and breezier too. Indeed, she no longer speaks to him as though she were conducting a BBC interview but only as a friend.

VICKI, **JACK**, and **MAX** appear exactly as before.

Setting: Inside JONATHAN's bedroom.

SCENE ONE

22ⁿᵈ May, 2001: *It is 5 p.m. The light-blue wallpaper inside
RICHARD and JONATHAN's double-sized bedroom is almost
completely covered with colourful posters of their favourite W.W.F
characters, including: Hulk Hogan, Big Boss Man, and Andre the
Giant. Cheap navy carpet covers the floor. A three-tiered unit -
packed to bursting with books accumulated since the boys' early
childhood - fills the entire left-side wall. Continuing clockwise, two
single divans rest against the main wall, opposite the door. Two white
bedside cabinets – topped with a black radio alarm clock; some
wrestling magazines; and a half-filled glass of water - divide them.
JONATHAN's bed is situated nearest the bay window, door right.
A large poster of his ever-favourite wrestler - the sinister looking
Undertaker - takes pride of place directly above his bed. A small,
bronze crucifix hangs on the side wall just above his pillow. Some
crisp-white netting and two pairs of mid-length, blue- mottled curtains
conceal the warped metal window frame. And a blue plastic box
containing JONATHAN's school books fills the tiny gap at the side
of his bed, beneath the bay window. A white Formica desk - stacked
with quality drawing pencils, a sketching pad, a small wooden
cross, some holy water, a statue of Saint Padre Pio and a variety of
medications - is awkwardly positioned at the foot of JONATHAN's
bed. Finally, two single wardrobes rest against the nearside wall, door
right. JONATHAN's wardrobe is significantly damaged from when
he once somersaulted off his bed and landed head first into one of the
doors. At the moment when filming begins, JONATHAN (wearing a
bright-yellow tee-shirt and black trousers) is sitting at the top end of
RICHARD's bed. CAROLINE is seated on a chair opposite him. To
her right, MAX is holding a fur-covered microphone into the air. And
to her left, just inside the open doorway, JACK is kneeling behind
his tripod and camera. Whilst VICKI (wearing a dark-grey hooded*

tee-shirt and light-grey trousers) is watching JONATHAN *on a small screen that has been set-up on the landing outside.* (*She speaks to camera*):

JONATHAN HASN'T SEEN ANY OF his friends since last Wednesday. Incredibly, he still hasn't told any of them how critically ill he is or even that he wears a prosthesis. Anyhow, because I reassured Jonathan that I would be home all evening he bravely went to Dean's house where he had arranged to spend a couple of hours with some of his closest mates. I dropped him off at around seven-thirty. However, when he unexpectedly telephoned home because he wanted to be collected much earlier than planned, he went simply crazy because I had nipped out to fetch Daniel from somewhere local. Naturally, I understood why he was so cross with me but I really hated seeing him so upset -

CARO (*tentatively*) It *is* different now that you've got … symptoms, isn't it?

JONATHAN Mmm.

CARO (*kindly*) I just really wanted to talk about that. How that felt for you and how you're coping with that 'cos …

JONATHAN Yeah. I know.

(*Pause*)

CARO (*still tentatively*) 'Cos it is … d … does it … ? (*Then much more directly*) Do you get frightened?

JONATHAN I get more frightened now because reality's kicking-in. (JONATHAN *takes a sharp intake of breath*) I just get more frightened about what's gonna happen. (*Pause*) 'Cos I knew things were gonna happen ever since the beginning (*he lightly sniffs*) … but then they were just far away … an' they seemed like … in the future … but now

134

they're kinda like drawing closer. (*Pause*) So I'm frightened 'cos now I've gotta start finking about 'em a bit more an' … just start getting prepared I s'pose. So … I'm getting a bit frightened in *that* sense.

CARO (*softly*) *What* are you frightened of?

JONATHAN Ermm, well … I dunno! It's just *how* it's gonna … how things are gonna come about and what warning signs am I gonna get and … yer know? (*Slight pause*) How mum's gonna take ev'ryfing. I'm really quite frightened for mum (*he lightly sniffs*) and the rest of 'em downstairs … more than me.

CARO (*gently*) But are you frightened of … pain, or are you frightened of dying?

JONATHAN (*clearly taken aback by* CAROLINE*'s extremely direct question*) Er, 'course I am, yeah. Mainly 'cos I don't know how it's gonna happen. I don't know … whether they're all gonna be around here when fings start to get really worse … or whether it's gonna happen unexpectedly, or … yer know? (*Pause*) So … I'm quite scared now … finking about it.

CARO But is it more about being frightened about *that* rather than what's coming after? *That* rather than …?

JONATHAN Sorry?

CARO (*quickly*) Do you feel quite kind of happy about … (*then more to herself*) Not happy, that's the wrong word, but …

JONATHAN I know.

CARO You know. You're actually scared of *how* it's gonna happen …

JONATHAN Yeah.

(*Together*)

CARO Rather than actually …

JONATHAN It's the … uncertainty of knowing about … *how* things are gonna come about that's … 'Cos, obviously, I know the ultimate: what's gonna … how it's gonna … eventually come about. But … it's just *how* it's gonna get there. I don't like finking about it really. I've actually … tried not to.

(*Pause*)

CARO (*softly*) *Do* you think about it? Does it …

JONATHAN Well, you can't help it! I mean … it's always trickling in the back of yer head but … trying not to let it *really* dominate. Although it's hard … it's always there.

CARO And I guess some people would say, you know, when you decided to have no chemotherapy, Jonathan … You've decided to have *some* treatment in the last week, haven't you?

JONATHAN That's radiotherapy, isn't it? It's completely different … to chemotherapy, though. I mean, obviously, I didn't accept chemotherapy 'cos … it's long-term …it's more drawn-out … and this radiotherapy's over a course of five days … and the side-effects is none. (*Pause*) You go up there. You have it. Lasts about five minutes. Then you can go home. You're not exactly admitted into hospital or anyfing. (*Pause*) You're not losing … your hair. You're not feeling sick. The only side-effects you get is … a bit of skin irritation. (*Pause*) So, I mean, it's completely different to … chemotherapy. Although it is *some* form of helpful treatment … (*then happily*) which is finished now anyway!

CARO And it was alright going in? Did it hurt when, you know, when you lay down in the dark? Did you think, "Ooh, this … ?"

JONATHAN No. Not really. Not at all.

CARO It's *not* scary?

JONATHAN No. It's just …what I thought it would be. (*Pause*) They don't *do* anyfing. They just … put this laser on you. You gotta lay there and … grin an' bear it for a couple of minutes … then it's all over.

CARO Was it hard having to go to the hospital every day for a week? 'Cos you have, for the last two months, been trying to avoid them.

JONATHAN Yeah … and I'm still trying to avoid them now!

CARO Sorry? You're trying to avoid what, Jon?

JONATHAN I'm trying to avoid going into hospitals 'cos … it's such a trek going up there and …it's just so many memories an' all that. So … going in there was … a bit of a … wasn't very nice but … luckily enough it was only for five minutes … so that's quite handy! But it's all over now … so I won't have to go up there for any more treatment.

CARO 'Cos have there been … ? Have they said to you they can do anything else to help you, treatment wise?

JONATHAN (*resignedly*) Well, it's now … just about the painkillers, innit? It's about … it's not about my shoulder or anymore lumps or anyfing … 'cos can't really get rid of them. So … now it's about pain control and (*he lightly sniffs*) … what kind of painkillers I can have. Combinations … of fings, yer know? (*Pause*) And how effective they'll be an' that's what I've been chewing over … with a couple of doctors today an' … (*now much quieter*) just about different … painkillers.

CARO And where does it hurt at the moment? What *is* the pain?

JONATHAN Now I can feel some kinda crackling. It's like some wheeziness in … in my back here (JONATHAN *leans forward and points to the centre of his back*). But I get … it all over really. Sometimes I get it there (JONATHAN *points to various parts of his back and chest*), there … an' sometimes I get a little bit of tightness there … where it's like forcing me *not* to breathe … where it's like I'm not allowed: I can't do it. It's like … when I breathe (JONATHAN *takes a sharp intake of breathe*) … it kinda stops an' there's no more room for air to go in. It's like a tightness … an' it's kinda frustrating. And it can be … quite painful as well.

CARO (*casually*) It must have been hard in the last two weeks to sort of face up to these things as being part of the cancer.

JONATHAN Yeah. Yeah. 'Cos I haven't … suffered from any of these symptoms. Remember when I saw Julian that day? I came home … and I was starting to get all breathless … and it kinda started to happen as soon as I saw him! And that came on *quite* quickly … I've gotta admit. (*Pause*) But, er, how quick things are gonna go now … I dunno. So … just gotta take fings as they come.

(*Pause*)

CARO Have you asked anyone how long?

JONATHAN I tried asking Julian about… how long it would take … and how quickly things would … come about, yer know, for me. But I fink … he knew what I was getting at. (JONATHAN *inhales deeply*) I think what he was saying was … *definitely* before the years out and … er, serious symptoms start to come maybe in a couple of months' time … or summink. I mean, ev'ryone's different ain't they? So … I'm really nervous about asking that. (*Pause*) But its summink … I feel I should ask him again actually. (*Pause*) Peace of mind and … security … stability in my mind knowing what's going on.

CARO (*gently*) He'd probably say he doesn't know, wouldn't he?

JONATHAN (*breathing deeply*) Well, I mean, he probably *doesn't* know … to be honest. He obviously doesn't know *exactly* when but … he must have a good idea … 'cos he sees it all the time, doesn't he? So I fink … he could give me a better idea than I've got at the moment. (JONATHAN *lightly sniffs*) But … I dunno. (*Now half smiling*) I'll ask him *later* rather than sooner. Postpone it a bit!

(VICKI *speaks to camera*):

I SUSPECT MY UNCONTROLLABLE NEED to monitor Jonathan during the night is the most likely cause of us both feeling constantly tired and irritable. It's true, when I accidentally wake him sometimes he gets *really* annoyed and shouts at me! But it's hard to sleep. Still, when he doesn't wake I often linger by his familiar bedside and pray for him, along with the rhythm of his irregular heartbeat that refuses to be silenced from inside his youthful chest. And yet, strangely, whilst I am painfully aware that Jonathan's untimely death will soon come to pass, I *always* feel especially blessed simply to have shared another day with him. Anyhow, I awoke this morning to the sharp, annoying sound of an incoming text message from our good friend Dee: *I'm sure the Holy Spirit will fill your hearts with the ability to cope during this difficult time* read her kind message. *So why do I feel so hopelessly sad?* I instantly replied. But Dee did not respond. Inconsolable, I promptly switched off my mobile phone and refused to look at it for the rest of the day -

CARO I mean, if things were offered to you to prolong … life for you, do you want that, or not?

JONATHAN (*quickly*) No! I don't. 'Cos that's what one of the discussions of chemotherapy … before … one of the possibilities was, "Oh, will it keep me here longer?" But it's all about the quality of life, innit? (JONATHAN *looks directly into* CAROLINE'S *eyes and speaks extremely openly and sincerely.*) And what quality of life would I have if … I'll *prolong* fings but … I'll be in bed. I won't be able to move! I'll be *so* sick … I won't be enjoying life, will I? (JONATHAN *takes a sharp intake of breathe*) There's just so many pros an' cons to weigh-up and … (*Pause*) I wouldn't accept anyfing anymore. No. Obviously I would if it was gonna help and if there was a chance but … (*softly*) there's no chances. It's gonna make me feel worse so … leave it.

Long pause. (VICKI *speaks to camera*):

I GREW *EXTREMELY* annoyed with Daniel and Rosie yesterday when they constantly bickered and argued together. Indeed, their inconsiderate behaviour only heightened my own intense stress knowing that Jonathan did not get the peace and quiet he so rightly deserves. Because, in truth, I sense his death is drawing closer by the day. I am permanently uptight. And scared. For everyone. Knowing the massive illusory time-bomb that was pre-set to shatter our whole world back in March, 1999, may actually explode at any moment. And as I brace myself, I am acutely aware that *all* of my children are looking to me for their strength and support but especially Jonathan. Oh, my God! *Please* don't let me fail them! -

CARO So the medication that you are on at the moment - is it only for pain control, Jonathan? Just so people understand that you *are* taking some of the things that Guy talked about, like steroids. They're different, aren't they? 'Cos some people don't understand that. I mean, you *are* on medication, aren't you?

JONATHAN Yeah. At the moment … I'm on codeine and paracetamol. It's like a mixture: kinda … take codeine two hours - paracetamol two hours. They're just painkillers (JONATHAN *lightly sniffs*) just to … help with the pain in my chest, obviously. (*Pause*) And I'm on steroids as well … which is like a treatment for anyfing really. It's not just for this. It's s'posed to be … helping the nerves, or summink, in my shoulder … 'cos I was getting pain in my shoulder so

… it's been helping that. But all the painkillers I'm on … it's nothing to do with the cancer or anyfing. Nothing can help that. It's just the pain. There's no, like … long-term treatment.

CARO (*softly*) Are you sleeping at night, Jon?

JONATHAN (*quietly*) Not really. No. I just stay awake some nights … thinking about fings, as you do. (*He sniffs loudly.*)

CARO (*gently*) What do you think about?

(*Pause*)

JONATHAN What's gonna happen. I mean … it's the same thing ev'ry night I fink about in my bed. (JONATHAN *mimics speech*) "Oh, *what's* gonna happen?" Yer know? You go through like a ritual in yer mind … before you go to sleep. Like how you fink things are gonna go and … how you'd like things to go in the circumstances.

(*Pause*)

CARO And *how* would you like it to be?

JONATHAN (*thoughtfully*) As peaceful as possible. As less fuss as possible. And as less pain as possible … really. I know there's gonna be *some* pain, obviously, but … (JONATHAN *half smiles at* CAROLINE) with as less as possible.

(*Pause*)

CARO And *where* do you want to be, Jon?

JONATHAN Here! In my bed. Don't wanna be … in hospital, or anyfing. I don't wanna be around people I don't know … and people that don't … don't, er, that don't really know me. I wanna be in my familiar surroundings … and that's where I *should* be.

CARO Have you talked about it to your mum?

JONATHAN Yeah.

CARO I mean, you've *actually* talked about …

(Together)

JONATHAN (*emphatically*) Yeah. Yeah.

Yeah, we have.

CARO Can you explain that to me? (*Pause*) *When* did you … was it a few days ago? Can you explain? Can you say, "My mum and I have talked about it".

JONATHAN What? My mum and I have talked about … where fings are gonna happen? Yeah. 'Cos she doesn't want me to be … somewhere else. Mum doesn't want me to be in … a hospital or anyfing. Obviously, she wants me to be in my home … and to spend as much time here as possible. Obviously. So it's lucky we both fink on those same lines … an' we both want the same things. (*Pause*) So I shall be here … (*quietly*) an' I won't be in no hospice.

CARO (*kindly*) *Why* don't you like the word 'hospice', Jon?

JONATHAN (*visibly cringing as he struggles to find the correct words that will best answer* CAROLINE*'s difficult question*) Oh! (*He then smiles at her.*) How do *you* know I don't like that word? (*Pause*) Oh, I dunno. It just reminds me of … yer know? It's depression, innit? I dunno. It's not a nice word! It's not as nice as 'home' is it? (*Jonathan smiles at Caroline, but this time more wisely.*) YOU know what I mean.

Pause. (VICKI *speaks to camera*):

JONATHAN AWOKE IN A UNUSUALLY depressed mood

last Sunday. And after much fuss, he eventually told me he did not sleep due to severe pain in his left leg. Concerned, I rang Flora straight away who advised me to give him two painkillers which made him exceptionally tired. Sadly, he became *so* sleepy that he was unable to welcome his dear cousin, Owen, who paid him an unexpected visit that same afternoon. Jonathan was truly disappointed about this. However, when he later told me that he had already taken some painkillers when I nipped to the shops earlier that morning, it was hardly any wonder he could not stay awake! Regardless, Jonathan's extreme downheartedness caused a strong wave of melancholy to wash over me too.

"Oh, well. That's the end of my social life!" Jonathan announced, when I entered his bedroom later that evening. He angrily nodded towards his left leg. Naturally, I tried to comfort him by saying his friends could always visit him at home. But he insisted: "That's *not* the same, Mum. You just *don't* understand!" And maybe he's right. Maybe it's impossible for me to fully understand what he is going through simply because I'm not the person who is dying from cancer. I'm just a desperate mum who wants no more than to help her sick child cope with the worst pain imaginable. In truth, knowing that I am unable to ease my beautiful boy's suffering in any way let alone save his life is killing me too. And this sad fact is causing irrepressible heartache that … -

CARO (*steadily*) So what's your priority now? Why *don't* you want to go and have treatment in a hospice? Can you explain? What do you wanna do over the next … however long?

JONATHAN (*clearing his throat, he takes a sharp intake of breath before he begins to speak*) I haven't got a plan. I haven't got a schedule, have I? (*Pause*) Got nothing to …

CARO But you said to me the other day, Jonathan … what you *really* wanted to do was to be normal, wasn't it?

JONATHAN Yeah, well … as normal as possible. Obviously, this isn't normal is it?

CARO Can you explain *that* to me then?

JONATHAN (*obediently*) Yeah. (*He takes another sharp intake of breath*) For however long I've got … I'd like to keep it as normal as possible - even though this isn't normal. But as normal … as you can be, I s'pose. (*Then very thoughtfully*) Yeah. Just go about fings … as yer would. (JONATHAN *lightly sniffs.*)

CARO What does normal mean in terms of your brothers and sister?

JONATHAN Normal? Well, I mean … being in hospital isn't normal … is it? Especially at this age. So it's about going about family life. (*Then much more quietly*) Obviously, I'll get limited as time goes on but, yer know … just keep going I s'pose.

CARO Would you give any advice to anyone else going through all this 'cos you're … What would you say?

JONATHAN I don't know if you *can* give advice …really. (*Very hesitantly*) I mean, people do their own fing 'cos you can't … this situation … you can't … people won't do what you tell 'em to do … 'cos it's too much of a serious subject. Too sensitive to go on other people's …: You can't say what's good for me is good for someone else 'cos it doesn't always work like that … does it? There are some people that *prefer* to be in hospital and be treated by nurses … and parents that wouldn't like the pressure of it all and yer know … want it to be in someone else's hands … and don't want the blame. So, you can't really give advice like that …I don't fink. (JONATHAN *lightly sniffs. Then emphatically*) That's what's good for *you*. And this is what's good for *me*. So it's what I'm gonna do.

Pause. (Vicki *speaks to camera*):

SECRETLY, AND TO MY UTTER amazement though, I cannot stop thinking about Jonathan's funeral. Obviously, I realise it would not be sensible to leave everything until the last minute just in case I'm unable to think straight when his time arrives. Because I want it to be perfect.

Anyhow, when Richard came home early from college last Friday he was visibly shocked to discover Jonathan using oxygen for the first time. In disbelief, he stared at his younger brother who was propped-up in bed wearing a plastic mask. Like a frightened rabbit, Richard shot straight out of their bedroom.

"I'm *really* scared, mum." He openly wept, when I caught up with him on the stairwell. Richard's heaving heart thumped loudly through his blue-cotton shirt. Huge tears rolled down his cheeks. I held him close.

"This is the hard bit, Rick." I gently told him. "But never forget: it's a lot worse for Jonathan than it is for us. So d'ya fink we could help each other out here?" Richard nodded. And through cloudy eyes, my eldest son and I made a secret pact to support each other as best we could through the coming weeks –

CARO (*gently*) And is your mum coping? (*She smiles warmly at* JONATHAN) 'Cos you *do* scrap a bit you two, don't you?

JONATHAN (*quickly*) That's family life, innit? *That's* what 'normal' is, innit?

CARO What is?

JONATHAN (*half smiling*) Arguing and, you know, 'scraping' … as *you* said. *That's* what being normal is. Ev'ryone argues … not *argue*

but, yer know, the occasional bit of banter going on. Ev'ryone has it!
So …

Pause. (VICKI *speaks to camera*):

SHOCKINGLY, THOUGH, THE THOUGHT OF Jonathan
dying no longer fills me with the same terror it once did. Because now,
whenever I look inside my beautiful boy's large, hazel eyes I can see
his life-spark is gradually fading with each passing day. Yes, for sure,
I know in my heart that my proud and fearless son is ready to die. So
now, whenever I pray I only ask God to release my cherished son from
his horrendous suffering and to quickly take him into heaven where he
surely belongs. And I *know* for certain that Jonathan is secretly praying
for this too –

CARO Would you say you're still enjoying life, Jon?

JONATHAN (*mockingly*) Enjoying!? Enjoying!? (*There is a long
pause whilst* JONATHAN *re-thinks* CAROLINE*'s unusual question*)
Well … I don't know about *enjoying*. No. I'm not enjoying … not
really. (*He half laughs*) How can you? I mean … not much to look
forward to … is there?

CARO But do you still get something from your days and your weeks?

(*There is another long pause*)

JONATHAN (*pensively*) Yeah. But it's *different*. There's no … .
Oh, I dunno!

(*Pause*)

CARO Are you glad you've got this time?

JONATHAN (*extremely positively*) Yeah. Of course I am, yeah. Yeah.
And I fink I'm lucky, I s'pose … that I know things aren't going to be

sudden and … yer know: one minute I'm here, one minute I'm not! (*Pause*) So at least I know I've got a bit of time to get my head around things … and people to get used to fings as well. Kinda count that as a blessing in a way. Got a bit of time knowing … (JONATHAN *lightly sniffs*), yer know?

CARO (*suddenly, but gently*) So how you gonna cope with your fear over the next few weeks? Is God helping?

JONATHAN (*frankly*) Perhaps. Yeah. Seems so.

(*Together*)

CARO (*persistently*) *Do* you feel closer to Him?

(*Pause*)

JONATHAN (*softly*) Yeah … s'pose.

CARO (*relentlessly*) But when you think about other people who haven't got religion, Jonathan, or don't believe in God … . That must be *really* hard.

JONATHAN I dunno where they'd be … to be honest. I dunno where *I'd* be … definitely.

CARO (*quickly*) Sorry? You don't know where you'd be if what?

JONATHAN I dunno where I'd be without religion … or anyfing. If I had nothing to … , yer know … look for. Even before all this started … I've always been the same. Even before I knew about all this. But I don't know where people would be if they didn't have anyfing. I just thank God I'm not in that situation.

(*Long pause*)

CARO (*quietly, and very respectfully*) Is there anything else you want to say, Jonathan?

JONATHAN Not if you've not got anyfing else on yer list.

(CAROLINE, JACK, *and* MAX *roar with laughter at* JONATHAN'*s humorous turn of speech.*)

CARO (*still half laughing, and in a highly exaggerated south London accent*) *ON* me list! Ain't there anyfing else! (*But* CAROLINE *soon returns to her usual professional self.*) (*Gently*) I don't know. What other things?

JONATHAN (*tiredly*) I dunno. I fink you've …

CARO I've covered the main things.

JONATHAN I fink you might have done, yeah. (JONATHAN *clumsily knocks into the large wooden picture frame that is hanging on the wall directly beside him.*) Oh! I keep knocking into that!

(*There is a long, uncomfortable pause.*)

CARO (*to* JONATHAN, *very softly*) Thank you. Thank you.

SCENE TWO

Sunday, 17th June, 2001: *It is 7 p.m. The bold, mid-summer sun is still shining brightly over* VICKI*'s small south London housing estate. Regardless, the vibrant purple and gold curtains inside her cosy bedroom remain tightly closed. The air is deathly silent. Everything is shrouded in a cloak of semi-darkness, including* VICKI*'s lifeless form which is completely hidden beneath her purple duvet. The white rosary beads are no longer entwined around the left bedpost. The purple teddy is lying face down on the floor. And the recently taken photographs of* JONATHAN *(seen in Act One) now adorn every inch of wall space inside this eerily quiet, yet peaceful, bedroom. The white chest-of-drawers are now positioned against the firmly closed door.* RICHARD, DANIEL *and* ROSIE *are on the landing outside. Whilst* JONATHAN *(wearing a bright-yellow shirt and black trousers) is seated at the foot of the bed. Presently, there is a soft knock on the bedroom door before* RICHARD*'s concerned voice is heard calling out to his mother. There is a long pause. Still silent,* JONATHAN *glides to the side of the bed and leans over* VICKI*'s buried form. She stirs a little when she feels several soft taps on her right shoulder. And when she hears* JONATHAN*'s familiar voice clearly calling to her in a firm, yet loving, manner her dishevelled head slowly emerges from beneath the duvet. There is another long pause. With great effort,* VICKI *(fully clothed in a short-sleeve, lilac blouse and black trousers) struggles to reach the side of her bed. The white rosary beads are loosely entwined around her pale fingers. And in her left hand, she is clutching a red school exercise book that she recently found in the blue box at the side of Jonathan's bed. She stares blankly at her dull reflection that is gazing back at her from inside the long mirror.* JONATHAN *calmly returns to the foot of the bed. He observes the critical way in which she is scrutinizing her swollen eyes; pinching her pale-grey cheeks; and tugging at her flat, dehydrated hair. Presently,* *there is another soft knock on the bedroom door. And* DANIEL*'s husky voice is heard calling out to his mother. Yet,* VICKI *– in a brisk and sloppy manner – mindlessly continues to remove the stale make-up off her sunken face.* JONATHAN *edges towards the closed window. Then, suddenly, as though hit by a bolt of lightning,* VICKI*'s grave expression switches into a look of sheer surprise and bewilderment. Still in semi-darkness, her excited eyes scan every inch of her bedroom in search for* JONATHAN. *At the same time, there is another soft knock on her bedroom door. And as* ROSIE*'s young, desperate cries are heard calling out to her mother,* VICKI *leaps onto her big brass bed; pulls back the curtains; and pushes open the stiffened windows. The remaining evening sunlight saturates the small bedroom. With equal speed, she moves the chest- of- drawers away from her bedroom door.* RICHARD, DANIEL *and* ROSIE *race towards her in a joyful manner.* VICKI *almost stumbles. But, thankfully, her children's outstretched arms soon support her. And as the happy group huddle together for a long time, they each fail to notice* JONATHAN *as he quietly disappears into the warm summer night.*

Scene closes to 'I Want to Vanish'
sung by Elvis Costello.

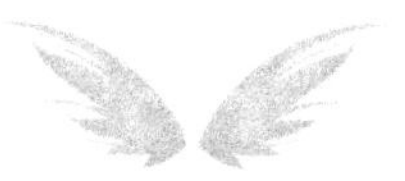

EPILOGUE

1

'The Promise'

6th June, 2001 (06.00 p.m.): IT WAS A BEAUTIFUL SUMMER'S
day. The air was hot and sticky. But not an inch of sunlight penetrated
the blue-mottled curtains that were tightly closed inside Jonathan's
teenage bedroom. Thankfully, the large electric fan situated at the foot
of his bed cooled us both. Indeed, its speedy hum also helped to ease
my pensive mind as I sat by Jonathan's familiar bedside regularly
smiling into his pale, young face each time he awoke in search of
my presence. Incredibly, at this time, I still believed my much loved
son would soon recover from his sharp decline in health especially
since Maureen – lead nurse from the Homecare Team - had visited us
much earlier in the day and kindly offered to sit with us for the entire
evening. Anyhow, with the loud, sonorous groan of Jonathan's heaving
chest; the hissing oxygen tank; and the humming electric fan all
resounding together inside my head, I lovingly observed my serene son
as he drifted in and out of sleep. We stayed this way for a long time.
Meanwhile, Daniel and Rosie were watching television downstairs.
Whilst Richard was busy representing Jonathan at the 'Do the Right
Thing' awards ceremony that was being held at our local town hall.

08.00 p.m: Jonathan suddenly awoke in a highly agitated
state. As Maureen attended to his pain relief, I fussed around him.
However, because Jonathan requested - much earlier in his treatment
- not to be heavily sedated at any time, I observed Maureen and the
careful way in which she used her professional judgement in a bid to
ease his obvious pain.

08.30 p.m: Both Maureen and I were astounded when Jonathan, once again, suddenly awoke. He was a lot more agitated than before. He was extremely hot too. He sweated profusely. In a desperate bid to cool him, I ran back and forth to the bathroom with a damp flannel which I routinely placed onto his burning forehead. At the same time, I noticed Maureen talking softly on her mobile phone. And as she paced the floorboards inside my tiny box-room, I intuitively knew that she was speaking to Simon from the Hospice about the amount of pain relief she had already administered. Anyhow, Jonathan's bony fingers tugged on his white-cotton tee-shirt that was now dripping with sweat.

"Shall I change it for you, darling?" I asked him, sympathetically.

Jonathan lightly nodded. But when he was unable to lift his arms above his head, I quickly found some scissors and carefully cut the tee-shirt straight off his back. With faces centimetres apart, I tenderly kissed Jonathan's warm cheek before whispering *I really love you* into his red-hot ear. Captivated by his intense gaze that always knew my thoughts and feelings, my serene son and I stared into each other's eyes for a long time. Overwhelmed, I almost stumbled when I recognised my own extreme sorrow mirrored inside Jonathan's own loving glare.

"Mum. I ... I ... give ... up." He feebly told me.

And I lightly nodded.

08.50 p.m: Turning the noisy oxygen tank onto its highest level, I dutifully held the plastic mask over Jonathan's young face until he had almost drifted back into another deep sleep. Then, to my dismay, he startled me once more when he unexpectedly sat bolt upright in a highly defiant manner. He appeared alarmed. And for a brief moment, I stupidly believed that God had finally answered my endless prayers for his speedy recovery. However, my childish optimism was soon dashed when another look of extreme anguish washed over him. Hurriedly freeing the plastic mask from his flushed face, Jonathan gasped in an extremely caring manner:

"Mum! *Please* ... don't ... grieve ... me ... for ... too ... long."

I was truly astonished.

"I'll try not to, Jonathan. I promise." I eventually spluttered.

Inconsolable from thereon, I freely wept beneath my beautiful boy's troubled gaze that was concerned only for me.

09.10 p.m: Richard innocently entered their bedroom in a light and breezy manner. Waving a fistful of brightly coloured cards into the air and grinning from ear to ear, he proudly declared:

"Hey, Jon! You won all of the top prizes tonight!"

Of course, Richard was totally unaware of Jonathan's current dilemma. But, thankfully, my half-turned back shielded him from his beloved brother's view. Without turning, I took a deep breath before calmly saying:

"Jonny's having some difficulties right now, Rick. Come back later."

Obediently, Richard's light footsteps tiptoed out of the room.

09.15 p.m: Jonathan's breathing grew even shallower. His heaving chest groaned louder. Worryingly, I noticed an unfamiliar look of fear inside his large, hazel eyes that I had never seen before. Scanning the room for Maureen's reassuring presence, I panicked when I could not see her. My shaky voice cried loudly into the semi-darkness:

"Maureen! Maureen! Jonathan needs you!"

Still holding the plastic mask over Jonathan's fearful face, I instinctively reached for his familiar hand and held it very tightly. And as our fingers entwined, I desperately willed my beautiful boy to stay with me for just a moment longer.

"You're doing *really* well!" Maureen cheerfully announced, when she finally re-entered the bedroom.

"That's … easy … for … you … to … say!" Jonathan bluntly wheezed back at her, from beneath his plastic mask. "It's … not … happening … to … *you*!"

Surprised, even slightly amused, by Jonathan's sharp response Maureen told him that she wholeheartedly agreed. Yet when she foolishly continued to praise him in the same over-confident manner, Jonathan gave her the most scornful look I have ever seen! Meanwhile, his breathing grew even shallower. Every nerve in my body twitched. And the solid lump inside my throat began to finally choke me.

09.20 p.m: Jonathan startled me once again when he suddenly became extremely aware of something outside of my own physical awareness. In a frantic manner, his large, hazel eyes scanned the bedroom:

"What's … all … that … noise? And … who … are … all … these … people?" He repeatedly asked me.

But when I told Jonathan that I could not see - or hear - anything unusual, he soon became even more alarmed. In truth, his sudden panic almost caused me to totally crumble. Yet, from somewhere, Jonathan found the strength to regain his usual dignified manner. And in that exact moment, we both knew our journey together was about to end. Our eyes locked. Our fingers tightened. I quickly sobbed:

"I *really* love you, Jonathan! I *really, really* love you!"

Jonathan's breathing grew much shallower. His strength was almost fully depleted. Then, to my utter amazement, he frantically freed the plastic mask from his troubled face and hurriedly gasped: "And I *really* love you too mum!"

09.25 p.m: I wept like a baby from thereon. I tenderly kissed Jonathan's familiar hand that was still clinging onto mine for dear life. Regardless, because my beautiful boy was clearly struggling to stay with me for as long as he could, I heard my own grief-stricken voice steadily say: "Go wiv the people, Jonny. Go wiv them now, darling; they've come to take you back to Jesus."

09.27 p.m: And as Jonathan continued to see and hear things outside of my own physical awareness, I continued to reassure him that it really was okay for him to leave me.

09.28 p.m: Then, gradually, Jonathan's heaving chest groaned no more. The air froze. I trembled. But still the noisy oxygen tank and the large electric fan hissed and hummed together for a long time inside my head.

2

MY GRIEF WAS ALL-CONSUMING in those early days after Jonathan's passing. I felt numb inside. My whole world stopped moving. I wept buckets. I shut myself away from family and friends, even my other children. Inconsolable, I placed the white-cotton tee-shirt that I cut off his back on the 6th June, along with his precious prayer cards and a small photograph of him beneath my pillow. I hoarded his personal belongings in suitcases beneath my bed. I clung to Ronan the Lion - his best childhood cuddly - as I cried myself to sleep each night wearing his favourite sweater that still had his smell on it. I continued to make him his early morning cuppa, routinely placing it on his bedside cabinet along with a usual ginger-nut biscuit. I even switched supermarkets because I could not stop my tearful eyes from searching out Jonathan's favourite foods. Furthermore, I raced to the cemetery every day to write him long, heartfelt letters which I always buried beneath the soil prior to leaving. Once, I became so engrossed in my own private thoughts that I failed to notice it was raining and also a full burial service had just taken place directly behind me! And on several occasions, because I could not sleep I drove to the cemetery in the dead of night simply to stare at Jonathan's fresh grave through the green metal railings that stood between us.

However, despite doing all these things my most comfort came from sitting beside a recent photograph of Jonathan that hung on my bedroom wall. There, I freely told his happy face just how much I loved him. And, on many occasions, I believe I heard my beautiful boy's familiar voice faintly responding: *I love you too, Mum!* And the light tingling sensation – as though a spider were running up and down the entire right-hand side of my body - only helped to convince me that Jonathan's spiritual presence was, indeed, sitting close beside me. But his soft, muffled tones that sounded like he was calling to me from inside a long tunnel never startled me. On the contrary, I always concluded my daily prayers by thanking God for the gift of Jonathan and asking Him to love and bless him wherever he may be.

3

29th June, 2001: WE CLEARED THE LOFT TODAY so it can be insulated before the winter months set in. It was quite a daunting task. But the busier I became, the less my anxious mind dwelled on Jonathan's recent passing. And as Richard ran up and down the rickety old step-ladder, I sorted through the piles of boxes, old handbags, and dusty bin-liners that were bursting with treasured memorabilia from our happy past.

The sharp, spiky-green branches of our old Christmas tree that once occupied an entire corner of our front-room for several years now bid us all a sad farewell. The disassembled pieces of an in-door baby swing that lovingly cradled my precious new-borns, now rattled and chimed beneath my busy feet. However, it was an unexpected find inside a large, candy-striped laundry bag that truly delighted me the most:

"Look kids! It's yer old books!" I shrieked with joy. Together, Rosie and I dropped onto the landing floor. "It's *Alfie, Annie Rose* and *The Tales of Trotter Street*!" I continued to rave.

"**And** *The Proud and Fearless Lion*!" Rosie innocently continued. "Wasn't that …?"

Instantly recognizing the jungle design with its proud protagonist lavishly sprawled across the front cover, I snatched Jonathan's favourite bedtime story out of Rosie's hand. Hot tears pricked my eyes.

"*The Proud and Fearless Lion.*" I quietly reminisced, just as Daniel came charging boisterously up the stairs.

"Can *I* help, mum?" he boomed, as the loft spat out yet another bulky bin-liner that landed only inches from our feet. Briskly standing, I brushed myself down.

"Okay, Dan. But don't ditch anyfing. Summa this stuff is very precious!" I told him.

"What! Like this *stupid* ol' fing?" declared Daniel, thoughtlessly dragging Rosie's christening gown out of a half-opened box.

"Blimey! Did I *really* fit into that! It's *so* tiny!" Gushed Rosie, sweetly.

"I know! 'ard to believe, ain't it? " quipped Daniel, grinning widely as Rosie's dark eyes suddenly filled with tears.

Anyhow, Richard eventually happened upon an old brown suitcase. Forgetting what it contained, I could hardly wait to open it! And yet, in all my haste, I was not quite prepared for the magnificent surprise that was about to unfold.

"Jonny would've hated all this dust!" remarked Richard, as he finally made his way back down the rickety old ladder.

"Yeah, bless 'im! He'd be sneezing all over the place!" I agreed.

Then, just moments later, we were all staring inside the old suitcase. Excitedly, I held Richard's first pair of grey school shorts high into the air. And we all roared with laughter when I retold how much he cried through his first year of primary school. Then I snatched-up Daniel's lemon and white baby-grow that lay close by: *Ahh, you looked so sweet in this!* I lovingly teased him. And, of course, Daniel, who was acutely aware of his deep dimples and the captivating power they still had over me, grinned very widely indeed. I smiled too.

Then I noticed a small, dark-grey box. It was half-hidden beneath a pile of multi-coloured children's clothes. I blindly opened it.

"Wow!" I screamed with delight. "It's Jonathan's first pair of baby shoes!"

Richard, Daniel, and Rosie grew instantly silent. Time froze. Unexpected tears rolled down my cheeks. They splashed onto the tiny red shoes that sat perfectly in the palm of my hand. The smooth leather still smelt divine. With the tip of my little finger, I traced the neat blue stitching that edged each sole along with the slight indents caused by Jonathan's teeny baby feet. A sharp pain ripped through my chest. I sobbed loudly. Then, within moments, I calmly returned Jonathan's first pair of baby shoes back inside their small, dark-grey box before quickly hoarding them beneath my bed along with *The Proud and Fearless Lion.*

4

7th February, 2018: LIFE WITHOUT JONATHAN HAS NOT been easy. He was a strong, loveable character and was especially endearing. In truth, not one day passes when I do not think of him. Sometimes I still cry for him too. But with the passage of time, I am now able to remember Jonathan in a much less painful way than I ever thought possible. Recalling our happier times together rather than the last few months of his life was the first step I took in helping me to control my overwhelming emotions. Because in those early days of bereavement, I forgot to remember that living with Jonathan was not all about living with cancer. Yet my healing could only begin once I learnt to focus more on the positive side of Jonathan's life instead of our last eighteen months together.

And yet, I do not expect to ever be pain free. Neither do I wish to be. Because somewhere entrenched in those bitter-sweet memories of Jonathan lay the deep-rooted bonds of love that we still share together wherever he may be. For sure, I know that these can never be erased simply because Jonathan's life experiences are also my own. And I do not wish to escape my past. It has shaped me. Anyhow, this book is a tribute to Jonathan's memory. It took me years to complete. And although it is an accurate account of his suffering, it is also a true testimony of the immense love and respect he held not just for his family and friends but also for his Christian faith.

Furthermore, writing this book proved to be the perfect antidote for my grief. It helped to heal me. But also during this time, I gained a BA Honours degree in English with Creative Writing; Richard and Rosie both qualified as primary school teachers; and Daniel as an electrician. Incidentally, Caroline and Jack married soon after completing their *Cancer* documentary. And the last I heard, they have a nice house somewhere in North London; are the proud parents of one boy and one girl; but, sadly, have still not managed to acquire that suitable garage!

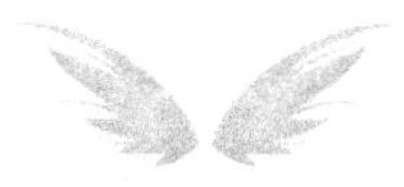

FINAL NOTE

Dear Reader, in Scene Four, Act Two it states: '…a red school exercise book …recently found in the blue box at the side of Jonathan's bed.' Here are the contents of that book.

'JONATHAN'S RED BOOK'

1

My hands were raised as I lay on my bed. I felt a spiritual presence nearby. I was in pain from my foot aching and could not sleep. I felt someone lay their hands on my head and I heard a deep voice mumble. I felt an amazing spiritual energy on my head – one like I've never experienced before. My head sank into my pillow and then I fell asleep. I woke-up and it was 8.30 a.m.

2

I was lying in bed when I felt a presence – an 'energy' (I always see a bright light when this happens.) I saw a man walking around my bed. He blessed my left side first. He walked around to my feet (I could hear his feet pattering) and he blessed my feet with his two hands. I was slightly frightened. He then blessed my left side again, then my right. With his head close to mine, and his hands over me, we both prayed (but I can't remember which prayer.) Then I saw my body from another angle. I watched the man as he pulled a ball of energy from my chest – my spirit! I then felt myself being lifted up – elevated – in his arms. We praised God. We 'flew' and ended-up somewhere else. The man crouched down and spoke to me but I cannot remember our conversation. As he began to leave, I watched him dancing and singing to God. I was crying tears of joy as I waved to him and said goodbye, not wanting him to go. I woke-up at 8.30 a.m.

3

My sleep was interrupted by the same powerfully strong light and spiritual energy. It lasted for about two minutes. I was blinded by it. Then, the same man (whom I now know to be Padre Pio) walked around my bed. I propped myself up onto my pillows and waited to see what he would do. He began by speaking to me about how our spirits can take us further than we can possibly imagine: "I know", I said. "You know?" "Yes", I said. "Good!" he proclaimed, "Because there IS a God!" He also said to me that people don't think that their spirits are important. Then we prayed a prayer that I was unfamiliar with. I awoke at 8.30 a.m.

4

I was dreaming that I was in church, kneeling and praying with my family. As I concentrated hard for another spiritual experience, I felt my spirit being 'thrown down' to the ground. I saw an angel. I was elevated again – seeing people beneath me. The angel carried me up through clouds. I heard a voice say to me, "Someday you'll be here!" Then I was kneeling in front of Jesus Christ, who was sitting on a high chair. The angel stood behind me. We prayed together. When we finished, the angel carried me back down again. I got brave and touched the angel on its back. It felt human. I woke-up at 8.30 a.m. I could feel

Jesus' presence in my room.

5

I got the light and energy again, as usual. An angel appeared to me. I said a few words but I cannot remember what they were. I awoke at 8.30 a.m.

(Same day, about 9.30 a.m.) This time I was fully awake, still lying in bed. The usual buzzing light and spiritual presence began. From the other end of the room, I heard Padre Pio's voice (as human as my own) say to me: "Hello people. This is Padre Pio – the one with the bleeding hands." He spoke in English with an Italian accent. He put his hands on my chest. I feel so holy and blessed.

6

I was in bed when I felt the usual light and energy. This time, there was a deep humming sound accompanying the light. I saw the figure of a little angel flying in front of me. There was little else for me to do, so I just watched him. Somehow, my hands were lifted as if I was praising God. I remember the angel showing me four pictures of people and I think one was of Mother Theresa. I could feel a hand holding my hand. I felt warm inside. When the angel went I woke-up and it was 6.30 a.m.

7

I said the 'Our Father' with Jesus. I heard His voice in my head, although I did not see Him. I awoke at 8.30 a.m.

8

I got the same feeling as I always get; a feeling that someone

*is over-powering my body. I saw the shadow of St. Therese's
head on the wall in front of me. It was surrounded by a bright
light. She was doing something to my back, which made it burn.
It was not a painful burn but if someone said to you: "FEEL
the Holy Spirit" then it would be this feeling. St. Therese was
saying some words in a French accent, "Oh, Jesus ..." she said,
and continued her prayer. "Give him ...", and I can't remember
the rest. She told me to "Get up" and "Escape". As she was
telling me to do this, I knew what she meant: escape from the
controlled feeling (anyone who has had this experience will
know what I mean). It took a struggle to get my head off the
pillow and everything felt strange – my pillow felt different.
"Excellent", she told me, as she guided me back down. I have
a feeling that she wanted me to look at her but I couldn't (not
that I didn't want to – I didn't have the energy). I remember
smiling when I heard her voice. This major experience has made
me forget other not so long experiences that also happened
throughout the night. I think she will be back. I wonder what
they want?*

9

*I felt the usual powerful light and presence. I knew what it was.
Then, I focused my attention to the end of my bed where I saw
Padre Pio. He had not even looked at me at this point. He was
looking at my statue of him; my pictures of Jesus and Mary; my
holy water; and other holy things that are on my desk. I saw him
bless them all with the sign of the cross. Then he looked at me
and walked up to me. I spoke first, saying: "Hello." He began
to laugh. I felt so comfortable around him. I still found it hard
to look at him because of his powerful presence. Then he said
to me: "Do you want to see me properly?" And I said, "Yes".
He put his hands over my eyes and about three seconds later he*

took them away. I remember saying: "Wow" and feeling happy. I could look at him without straining. I had never been so happy to see him. This time it seemed like he was visiting as a friend. He asked if there was anything I wanted to say to him and so I asked: "Did St. Therese really visit me last night?" He said, "Yes". I don't know why I asked that question because I am so sure she did anyway (I whispered the question into his ear). I remember talking and laughing a lot. He was so happy. When he went he said, "Goodbye" and went out through the door. I awoke at 8.30 a.m.

10

My eyes were open but I was feeling all the same feelings again. My attention was focused on a picture of Jesus in front of me. I definitely felt a presence. I made the sign of the cross and felt it more. It lasted about five minutes. From the 'Divine Mercy' picture (on my desk) there came a power; a light; an energy.

11

I was dreaming when suddenly my dream turned into something. I began to feel so holy and spiritual. The same 'energy', light and power that I have mentioned before were all involved. I felt my body 'turn' so that I was facing ahead. I saw a female figure holding a picture in front of her face (the picture was of her and I am almost sure it was St. Therese again). I lifted my hand up to touch her but I came to a point where I couldn't go any further. The same was felt with my left arm reaching out. I began crying happy tears. I was not 100% sure who it was.

12

I was asleep when all of a sudden I got the usual feelings of power around me: white light and a spiritual feeling in my heart. I remembered Father Michael telling me to pray the next time it happens, so I said the 'Lord's Prayer' and the 'Hail Mary'. In front of my bed is a picture of Padre Pio and in this picture I could recognise his hands with gloves on. The picture was acting almost like a mirror because when I lifted my hands I could see them reflecting in the picture. It seemed to last for a long time. I touched his hands and they felt so real. As I touched his hands the feeling I got was unbelievable. I awoke at 6.30 a.m.

13

I was in bed and saying a prayer to St. Therese in a sleepy state. I can't remember what the prayer was but after I had said it she appeared to the left of me. I was over-powered with the usual feelings of an incredible spiritual presence. At first, I thought it was Padre Pio but then I heard a voice say, "Hello". It was a French female's voice and then I knew. I was talking but I don't know how loud because I was hearing the 'humming' of the powerful presence. I said, "Hello, did you hear me?" meaning did she hear my prayer. Laying her hands over me she said, "I realised you needed me."

This is the last entry Jonathan wrote in his RED BOOK. I feel honoured that he spoke to only me about them, along with other similar spiritual experiences which occurred regularly and throughout the last twenty-eight months of his life. I'm positive they went a long way in helping him to accept his untimely death. I truly believe it to be so.

www.ingramcontent.com/pod-product-compliance
Lightning Source LLC
Chambersburg PA
CBHW051451050726
47593CB00005B/2028